OVER DOSE

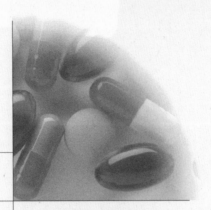

Over

The Case Against

Jeremy P. Tarcher/Penguin
a member of Penguin Group (USA) Inc.
New York

Jay S. Cohen, M.D.

Dose

the Drug Companies

Prescription Drugs,
Side Effects, and Your Health

Most Tarcher/Penguin books are available at special quantity discounts for bulk purchase for sales promotions, premiums, fund-raising, and educational needs. Special books or book excerpts also can be created to fit specific needs. For details, write Penguin Group (USA) Inc. Special Markets, 375 Hudson Street, New York, NY 10014.

Jeremy P. Tarcher/Penguin
a member of
Penguin Group (USA) Inc.
375 Hudson Street
New York, NY 10014
www.penguin.com

First trade paperback edition 2004
Copyright © 2001 by Jay S. Cohen, M.D.

The Library of Congress cataloged the hardcover edition as follows:

Cohen, Jay S.
    Over dose : the case against the drug companies : prescription
drugs, side effects, and your health / by Jay S. Cohen.
        p.   cm.
    Includes index.
    ISBN 1-58542-123-5
        1. Drugs—Side effects.   2. Pharmaceutical industry.   I. Title.
    RM302.5 .C64   2001   2001027737
    615'.1—dc21
    ISBN 1-58542-370-X (paperback edition)

Printed in the United States of America
10 9 8 7 6 5 4 3 2 1

Book design by Tanya Maiboroda

To my family, friends, and colleagues for their years of support and encouragement for this work. And to the many patients who extended their trust and shared their stories with me.

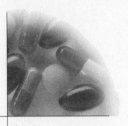

Acknowledgments

QUALITY WORK REQUIRES quality people, and I have been blessed with many in the creation of this book. First and foremost is Barbara, my wife of twenty-two years, who has proofread every version of every draft of every chapter of this book for three years. Paul Lapolla has been not only my agent, but also a major force in helping shape the book, and a friend who was always available to discuss the project, or politics, or any aspect of life itself. Mitch Horowitz is the experienced, intelligent, accessible, down-to-earth editor whom every writer wishes for but few have. Jeremy Tarcher is the first publisher who bothered to discuss a book personally with me and to make himself accessible throughout the publishing process. David Korzenik provided an insightful tutorial on the legal issues involved with controversial topics.

Through all the years of research and writing, and despite poor health and tough times, Barbara, my son Rory, my mother Delores Levy, stepfather David Levy, and other family members have been consistently caring and supportive. Barbara Slater, the chief librarian at the University of California Biomedical Library, has been an invaluable source of assistance, encouragement, and wit. My department chairmen, Bob Kaplan in Family and Preventive Medicine and Lewis Judd in Psychiatry, have also been constantly supportive of my research. To all of these people, I express my deep thanks and appreciation.

Author's Note

THE PURPOSE OF THIS BOOK is to help readers become more informed consumers of medical services and prescription drugs and to assist them in consulting more effectively with their own physicians. The use of prescription medications can be directed and managed only by a doctor. The information in this book should not be treated as a substitute for the direct medical advice of a doctor. Readers should not change drugs or dosages unless specifically directed to do so by their own doctors.

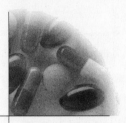

Contents

Table of Figures

Over Dose

Chapter 1

The Race to the Bottom

I WAS IN MY RECLINER, headset on, writing this book, when the telephone rang.

"Dr. Cohen, my name is Alex. I'm sorry to bother you, but I need to speak to you about problems I'm having with my medication."

I don't get many calls. After twenty years in practice, I've been disabled for ten. I have no office or funding for my research, so I work at home. My telephone number is unlisted. Alex, a young man from the other end of the country, had obviously gone to considerable trouble to find me.

"I'm taking Prozac for panic attacks and depression," he told me. "I was nearly housebound by agoraphobia once. I was okay for three years, but things got stressful at work and the problems returned."

"Prozac is a reasonable choice for your disorder," I said. "What's the problem?"

"I've gotten much worse since starting the drug. I get terribly agitated now, and my heart pounds and I can't sleep. I get so shaky some-times, I'm afraid to go out. I'm withdrawing and depressed again. I think the Prozac is making me worse."

"What do your doctors say?"

"They say that the side effects from the Prozac—the insomnia and palpitations—show that it is working, and that I should wait it out."

I sighed quietly. This was awful advice, but not unusual. Although I already knew the answer, I asked, "What dose of Prozac are you taking?"

"Twenty milligrams a day."

Twenty mg—that's what Eli Lilly and Company, Prozac's manufac-turer, recommends initially for otherwise healthy people aged eigh-teen to sixty-five, and that's what physicians prescribe. Unfortunately, neither Alex nor his physicians knew that early research had already shown that doses one half or even one quarter Lilly's recommended amount are all that some patients need.[1,2] Anything greater com-monly causes side effects including agitation, insomnia, rapid heart rate, and consequent depression and social withdrawal. These are signs that Alex was being overdosed.

Alex isn't alone. In 1998 an extensive study published in *The Jour-nal of the American Medical Association* (*JAMA*) showed that 106,000 people die annually in American hospitals from medication side ef-fects.[3] Medication reactions are the fourth leading cause of death in the United States, dwarfing the number of deaths caused by automo-bile accidents, AIDS, alcohol and illicit drug abuse, infectious dis-eases, diabetes, and murder. In addition to the medication-related deaths, the *JAMA* study also tallied 2,216,000 severe medication reac-tions in U.S. hospitals annually.

Because of the especially rigorous methods the researchers ap-plied, even these numbers may not present the full picture. The au-thors defined serious side effects narrowly, including only clear-cut reactions causing permanent disability, hospitalization, or death. Thus, they excluded side effects that disable people for weeks or months, side effects such as dizziness or sedation that cause automo-bile accidents or falls and broken limbs, side effects that require emergency interventions, and side effects that prolong hospitalizations or force people to miss work. And the authors didn't even try to count the largest category of all: side effects occurring in outpatients. Overall, they excluded side effects that occur far more often than the ones they included.

Despite omitting so many side effects, the *JAMA* study still recorded numbers reaching epidemic proportions. And, as the authors noted, this side-effect epidemic wasn't new: "The incidence has remained stable over the last 30 years."[4]

BECAUSE IT IS sometimes difficult to place such statistics in everyday terms, consider this: 106,000 deaths a year averages out to nearly 300 deaths a day, *every day*. In comparison, about 85 people died from accidents linked to faulty Firestone tires. The Firestone deaths occurred over a period of several years; medication reactions kill 300 people every day. Yet it was the Firestone deaths that dominated the news for several weeks and drew Congressional hearings.

Deaths from all major airline crashes in the United States average less than 300 annually, but one airplane crash gets more media attention and governmental scrutiny than the 300 medication-related deaths that occurred not only the same day as the airline crash, but also every day before and after for decades.

Why has this epidemic of side effects gone unrecognized? Deaths from medication reactions rarely look any different from natural deaths. There's no visible wreckage to videotape, no crash sites to horrify and fascinate viewers. As media people say, "No film, no story." Medication deaths often occur quietly in hospitals, emergency rooms, and homes. When medication-related deaths occur, it is often unclear at first whether the cause was the medication, the illness, or other factors. In other words, to much of the media, there's nothing sexy about side effects.

Moreover, the public likes to believe that our hospitals and medications are safe and that our doctors are taking every reasonable precaution. Facing the failure of a major industry is never comfortable. How many decades did it take to recognize the drunk-driving prob-

4

lem? To bring the dangers of cigarettes to public awareness? To mandate seat belts in cars? Maybe with medication side effects it's the same: We'd rather not know.

IT MIGHT BE different if the public received an accurate account of the scope of the side-effect epidemic. Alex's experience, for example, may have been severe enough to drive him to contact an unfamiliar doctor 2,500 miles away, but his case will never be counted in the side-effect statistics. His doctors didn't recognize Alex's side effects, and even if they had, they probably wouldn't have reported them to the Food and Drug Administration (FDA). "Most physicians feel that detecting adverse reactions is a professional obligation, but relatively few actually report such reactions [to the FDA]," states *Goodman and Gilman's The Pharmacological Basis of Therapeutics,* one of medicine's most respected drug references.[5] Dr. Brian Strom, former chairman of the department of biostatistics and epidemiology at the University of Pennsylvania, told *The New York Times* in 1997: "Most doctors don't know the system [for reporting medication reactions to the FDA] exists."[6] When speaking to medical groups, Dr. Strom shows a slide of an FDA MedWatch form and asks: "How many of you have ever seen that?" Usually, less than a third raise their hands.

Yet, it is from voluntary reports from physicians that side-effect statistics are derived. Physicians, however, often feel that so-called minor side effects—the ones that make millions of people like Alex feel merely miserable or unable to function normally—aren't worth reporting. Reporting more serious reactions may raise questions about treatment or lead to lawsuits. Another highly regarded drug reference, *Melmon and Morrelli's Clinical Pharmacology: Basic Principles in Therapeutics,* comments: "Drug-induced complications can mimic and therefore be attributed to disease-induced problems. When therapy fails, we [physicians) frequently can attribute the failure to the disease and escape blame. Probably nowhere else in professional life are mistakes so easily hidden, even from ourselves."[7] The result is that only one in twenty side effects is reported to authorities.[8,9]

Drug companies and medical institutions have their own reasons for underestimating the full scope of the side-effect epidemic. Dr. David Bates, an associate professor of medicine at the Harvard Medical School, wrote in *JAMA*:

Hospitals have had strong incentives not to identify too many of these adverse drug events. Reporting large numbers of adverse events and any serious preventable event brings intense scrutiny from regulators and the public. Thus, most hospitals have relied on spontaneous reporting, which only identifies about 1 in 20 adverse reactions and leads to the perception that injuries from ADRs are less common than they really are.[10]

Even the FDA acknowledges that adverse drug reactions are grossly underreported. In March 2000, *Dickinson's FDA Review* reported on its interview with Jerry Phillips, associate director of the Office of Post-Marketing Drug Risk Assessment at the FDA:

These reports, however, are generally believed by experts to grossly understate the actual situation, Phillips said. In the broader area of adverse drug reaction data, the 250,000 reports received annually probably represent only 5% of the actual reactions that occur.[11]

A simple extrapolation from these numbers reveals a total of five million medication reactions each year—and this is still probably an underestimate.

However, one by one, the public is learning about the perniciousness of the side-effect epidemic. Knowledgeable people have told me that their elderly parents died not from their illnesses but from being prescribed too many too powerful medications. Dozens of Web sites now exist where patients can discuss medication reactions that have caused major reactions or disabilities that their physicians have ignored. Many physicians dismiss anecdotal reports or cases posted on the Internet, but scientific discovery often begins with individual reports of an unrecognized or poorly understood problem. These reports, especially when hundreds of in-depth, medically credible descriptions are listed, should be taken seriously, because they represent another unrecognized aspect of the side-effect epidemic.

IT MIGHT BE different if the side-effect epidemic were caused by a few bad drugs. Every industry produces some lemons. Thus the FDA has had to remove ten prescription drugs (plus a vaccine and an anesthetic) within the last four years. But, as this book will document, the problem extends well beyond these few. Instead, it involves hundreds of drugs including top-sellers like Viagra, Premarin, Prozac, Lipitor, Celebrex, and Motrin. Because the problem is so large and so many drugs are involved, blame is difficult to assess. In addition, these same drugs help millions of people, which further obscures the many problems they cause, why they cause them, and how easily many of these side effects, like Alex's, can be avoided.

Consider, for example, one class of medications: women's hormones. When I was a medical intern in 1971, I treated a young woman with a blood clot in her lower leg (thrombophlebitis). She required hospitalization and bed rest for nearly two weeks. She was lucky: Hundreds of women like her died each year when such clots broke free and coursed to their lungs. These clots were caused by birth control pills—pills that in the 1960's and seventies contained three to eight times more estrogen and progesterone than actually needed.[12] That's 300 to 800 percent more of these powerful hormones than today's pills—doses that exposed millions of women to greatly increased risks of blood clots, strokes, and death. The death rate from thromboembolism alone was 600 percent higher with the original high-dose pills. I don't know where my patient is today, but probably she is now worrying about the increased risks of breast cancer that have been reported with these high-dose pills.[13-16] How many women have been harmed by these excessive doses that were prescribed in the United States for twenty-eight years? Some data exist, but the full extent of the damage has never been defined.

Perhaps my patient, after entering menopause, received hormone therapy for hot flashes. If she was prescribed Premarin for hot flashes at the dosage recommended by its manufacturer, Wyeth-Ayerst, she might have received double or even quadruple the amount she actually needed. Wyeth-Ayerst recommended 1.25 mg of Premarin as its initial dose for hot flashes from 1954 through 1999, long after medical experts had shown that 0.625 mg and even as little as 0.3 mg were sufficient for many women.[17–19] Premarin is perhaps the most prescribed drug ever; in 1999 alone, women purchased more than 47 million prescriptions in the United States. Yet even in 2000, after Wyeth-Ayerst finally reduced its recommended starting dose for hot flashes to 0.625 mg, this amount remains excessive for some women.[20–22] Similarly, the recommended doses of Premarin for preventing osteoporosis have been unnecessarily high for many women.[23,24] Meanwhile, estrogens like Premarin have been linked to increased rates of breast cancer[25,26]—and it is likely that the higher the dose of estrogen, the greater the risk. Has my patient been affected? How many thousands of women have been harmed over the years? We'll never know, and the side-effect statistics will never reflect them.

Why weren't lower, safer, effective doses of these hormones, as used today, developed decades earlier? The technology existed in the 1960's to determine the lowest, safest doses of these potent drugs. But the intense, fast-paced competition of the medication marketplace frequently spurs drug companies to conduct small, brief, insufficiently extensive studies on the dosages of new drugs[27]—dosages that will be taken by millions of people. The result is that only belatedly, years or even decades later, do we discover that lower doses are not only effective, but avoid many side effects. Of course, by this time, tremendous damage has been done to people and their families.

The story is the same with many drugs—not just obscure drugs, but many top-selling drugs. The problem encompasses the entire field of medication therapy, as recognized experts have attested:

• Carl Peck, M.D., former director of the FDA's Center for Drug Evaluation and Research: "There are noteworthy examples in drug development of failing to get the dose right when a drug is first marketed."[28]

- Dr. Raymond Woosley, the chairman of the department of pharmacology at Georgetown: "The U.S. society has invested in developing wondrous new pharmacologic therapies but has failed to invest adequately in their safe use."[29]
- Dr. Norman Sussman, editor of *Primary Psychiatry:* "There are lots of problems with the current system of drug testing. Often it fails to detect efficacy and, more often than would be desired, misses significant side effects."[30]
- Dr. Marcia Angell, former editor-in-chief of *The New England Journal of Medicine:* "To rely on the drug companies for unbiased evaluations of their products makes about as much sense as relying on beer companies to teach us about alcoholism."[31]

The result of these shortcomings? Dr. Thomas J. Moore of Georgetown University, Dr. Bruce Psaty of the University of Washington, and Dr. Curt Furberg of Wake Forest University determined that "51% of approved drugs have serious adverse effects not detected prior to approval."[32] Think about this: More than half of our drugs, after being deemed "safe" by the FDA and then prescribed to millions of people, are subsequently detected to have previously unrecognized, medically serious side effects. No wonder we have a side-effect epidemic.

WHEN THE MAJORITY of our drugs are approved with serious risks, the threat isn't small. Forty-six percent of Americans take at least one prescription drug daily.[33] That's more than 128 million people. Most of these people are taking medications long-term, so their exposures aren't brief. Twenty-five percent of Americans take multiple prescription drugs every day. In 1999, Americans purchased 2,587,575,000 prescriptions: That's nine prescription drugs (as well as several over-the-counter drugs) for every person in America.

Americans paid $125 billion for these prescriptions—$50 per prescription on average. One would think that with so much cost and utilization, medications would be our most carefully manufactured and safest products. Yet, as Dr. Bates wrote: "Only after drugs leave the trial setting and are used in sicker patients do their true risks become apparent."[34]

It doesn't have to be this way. As Dr. Bates also wrote, "Although some risks are inevitable, they can be significantly reduced."[35] I agree: Side effects can be significantly reduced, but they aren't. The inadequate methods by which drugs are developed and prescribed are why.

Weary of seeing avoidable side effects affect patient after patient, I began investigating the origins of this problem. With a background in general medicine, pain research, general pharmacology and psychopharmacology, and experience as a staff member at UCLA, UCSD (the University of California, San Diego), and at the world's largest naval medical center at Balboa Hospital in San Diego, I began voicing my concerns publicly in 1988. First I wrote letters to medical journals and authored health columns in a local newspaper. Beginning in 1996, I began publishing lengthy articles describing my findings in respected medical journals such as the *Archives of Internal Medicine*,[36-38] *Postgraduate Medicine*,[39] *Geriatrics*,[40] *The Annals of Pharmacotherapy*,[41,42] and *Drug Safety*.[43]

After more than a decade of research conducted without any influences, I found that the drug companies dominate the entire process of medication therapy—from early research to ultimate usage—as few other industries control their products today. Drug company research and development often serves marketing strategies more than sound science or patients' safety. The many ways that drug companies accomplish this is discussed in depth in Chapter 9, but here is a glimpse—derived from numerous medical journal articles, including *JAMA*,[44] *The New England Journal of Medicine*,[45] and *Lancet*,[46]—of the methods that drug companies use in accomplishing their goals:

- Drug companies can choose research study designs that are more likely to produce favorable results rather than designs that may provide more accurate results.
- Drug companies can conduct multiple studies on new drugs, then select and publish the most favorable ones while suppressing the rest.

- Drug-company studies can measure a drug's effectiveness in multiple ways, then select and publish only the best results. Sometimes these favorable results have little to do with whether the drug will help patients.
- Drug companies hire professional writers to prepare articles according to company guidelines, using favorable phrases and terms selected by the companies.
- Drug companies hire high-profile experts to place their names on drug-company-generated articles, although the experts have not participated in the studies and their financial connections with the drug companies are not disclosed.

These excesses might be unimportant if drug-company research represented a small portion of all medication research. However, the drug companies underwrite 70 percent of all medication research today.[47] This gives the pharmaceutical industry tremendous power over the entire medication research effort, including the threat of lawsuits or loss of future funding for physicians wanting to publish unfavorable findings.[48] More and more, drug companies are requiring researchers to sign confidential agreements before receiving any funding, giving the companies the power to suppress findings they don't like.

The pharmaceutical industry's ability to amass wealth while hospitals and medical centers struggle financially has allowed the drug companies to intrude into the arena of independent academic medicine.[49] This intrusion is so great that in 2000, Dr. Angell issued an astonishing article—"Is Academic Medicine for Sale?"—in *The New England Journal of Medicine:*

Academic medical institutions are themselves growing increasingly beholden to industry. . . . Some academic institutions have entered into partnerships with drug companies to set up research centers and teaching programs in which students and faculty members essentially carry out industry research. . . . When the boundaries between industry and academic medicine become as blurred as they now are, the business goals of industry influence the mission of the medical schools in multiple ways. . . . The influences of the marketplace should not become woven into the fabric of academic medicine. We need to remember that for-profit businesses are pledged to increase the value of their investors' stock. That is a very different goal from the mission of medical schools.[50]

Despite the concerns of Dr. Angell and other experts, drastic reductions in insurance and Medicare payments have placed great pressure on medical institutions and research physicians to accept the money—and terms—of the drug companies. At the same time, the drug companies spend billions targeting office physicians, as well as new interns and residents, with gifts, free meals, travel subsidies, and subsidized symposia presenting the drug companies' spin on their medications.[51,52]

Beyond these direct influences, drug companies exert broad influence over the drug information received by doctors and consumers. The vast majority of everything physicians and consumers read and know about medications comes from the drug companies. Medication package inserts, drug advertising toward physicians and consumers, and the information in the ubiquitous *Physicians' Desk Reference* (*PDR*)[53] come directly from the drug companies. Where do most doctors turn for medication and dosage information? To the *PDR*, to drug company representatives who make the rounds of doctors' offices, and to advertising in medical journals. Yet, the medication information offered by these drug-company-supported sources is often biased, incomplete, and sometimes inaccurate.

The *PDR* is not only the leading drug reference among physicians, but it is also purchased by thousands of consumers each year. Moreover, the *PDR* is the source for the bulk of information contained in other consumer drug references. However, as I have written in multiple professional publications, because the *PDR* is mainly a collection of drug-company-written package inserts, it omits a great deal of important information. The *PDR* omits or underreports many serious side effects. It frequently omits information about proven-effective medication dosages that are lower and safer than the doses recommended by drug companies or usually prescribed by doctors.[54–58] Many new, important uses of medications are not even mentioned in the *PDR*. Nor does the *PDR* provide any guidance whatsoever in selecting between the many drugs that might be used for medical conditions. And, although a new *PDR* is published each year, many drug descriptions are not updated. Some of these descriptions contain information that is decades old.

A glaring example was provided in a 1997 article in the *Annals of Emergency Medicine*.[59] This article examined drug-company guidelines in the *PDR* for handling overdoses of twenty drugs commonly seen in overdose situations in emergency rooms. The study found that for 80 percent of the drugs studied, the *PDR* guidelines for handling overdoses were inadequate. For overdoses with nearly half of the drugs, the *PDR* recommended "ineffective or frankly contraindicated" treatments that could worsen the situations or cause unnecessary deaths.

THE DRUG COMPANIES' influence even extends to the FDA, which we will explore in Chapter 11. The FDA is required to ensure the effectiveness and safety of medications, but changes in the law and political pressure from Congress, as well as a massive shortfall in funding, has led to weakened FDA standards. Furthermore, some of the FDA's own policies make matters worse.[60]

Funding for the FDA's monitoring of newly approved drugs is so limited that some drug toxicities weren't identified by the agency but by investigations conducted by newspapers or health interest groups. Limited funding also hampers the ongoing monitoring of important drugs with recognized risks. After Viagra was on the market for seven months, the FDA reported receiving 230 cases of deaths associated with the drug.[61] The FDA responded, as usual, with required changes in Viagra's labeling—yet, the agency hasn't provided any follow-up reports on Viagra-related deaths or any analysis of whether the labeling changes have helped.

Experts with drug-company ties fill many important advisory positions at the FDA. An investigation by *USA Today* found that more than half of the experts on FDA advisory committees "have financial relationships with the pharmaceutical companies that will be helped or hurt by their decisions."[62]

Today, the FDA approves drugs much faster, and sometimes on fewer studies, than required ten years ago,[63–65] and FDA oversight wasn't exactly robust then, as multiple drug withdrawals in the 1980's demonstrated. Since 1997, more drugs have proven toxic and been withdrawn than ever before. Some of these withdrawn drugs—Redux, Seldane, Propulsid, Rezulin—were prescribed millions of times. According to Dr. Alastair J.J. Wood, Assistant Vice Chancellor for Research at the Vanderbilt University Medical Center, "a staggering 19.8 million patients (almost 10 percent of the U.S. population) were estimated to have been exposed" to just five of the ten drugs withdrawn in this period.[66] Dr. Wood added, "None of the drugs was indicated for a life-threatening condition nor, in many cases, were they the only drugs available for that indication."[67] Safer alternatives to these drugs existed, but intense marketing convinced physicians to prescribe them anyway—and to continue prescribing them even as the FDA prepared to withdraw them.

Drug companies can profit handsomely on such drugs. Seldane, the top-selling antihistamine in the world for more than a decade, was on the market for thirteen years until the FDA removed it in 1997, seven years after the drug's cardiac toxicities were identified in 1990.[68] Perennial top-seller Propulsid, for heartburn, remained on the market for seven years, despite reports of hundreds of heart arrhythmias and scores of deaths before the FDA finally withdrew it.[69] Rezulin, a diabetes drug withdrawn by Britain in 1997, wasn't withdrawn by the FDA until 2000, during which hiatus Warner-Lambert earned $1.8 billion.[70]

Drug-company influence on regulatory agencies isn't solely an American affair. "Some medicines are out on the market too early, without giving practitioners sufficient time to evaluate them," Dr. Thiery Buclin, a Swiss health official, told *Dimanche*, a leading French newspaper, in April 2000. "We have proof of too much hastiness and sometimes lack of prudence. In 1998 alone, out of thirty medicines launched in the Swiss market, five had to be removed. This is a significant number of rejects, revealing a counter-productive mechanism. The pharmaceutical industry plays the first role in this dangerous game. With aggressive marketing, it uses heavy infantry to convince health personnel."[71]

Aggressive marketing, slanting research, unethical publishing of results, pressuring medical centers, intimidating researchers, influencing physicians, limiting information, manipulating the FDA, marketing drugs with inaccurate safety information and inappropriate doses—all of these have created an environment in which medication development has become, in Dr. Angell's fitting term, a "race to the bottom."[72]

THE SIDE-EFFECT epidemic arises from the very methods by which drugs are produced, and thus it involves hundreds of medications. That's why warnings like this *partial sampling* from January 1998 to January 2000 continue to appear in medical journals and the news media:

- "Correctly Prescribed Drugs Take Heavy Toll: Millions Affected by Toxic Reactions."—*Washington Post*[73]
- "Lawmakers Ask FDA Why Rezulin Was Kept on Market Despite Deaths."—*Los Angeles Times*[74]
- "Hepatotoxicity Associated with Antiretroviral Therapy in Adults Infected with HIV."—*Journal of the American Medical Association*[75]
- "Some AIDS Patients Are Hit by Disfiguring Fat Deposits; Protease Inhibitor Drugs Suspected."—*Philadelphia Inquirer*[76]
- "Sudden Deaths Reported with Orap."—*Worst Pills, Best Pills News*[77]
- "Alcohol-Acetaminophen [Tylenol] Syndrome: Even Moderate Social Drinkers Are at Risk."—*Postgraduate Medicine*[78]
- "Psychosis Due to Abrupt Discontinuation of Oral Contraceptive."—*Primary Psychiatry*[79]
- "Antibiotic Linked to Stomach Disorder in Infants."—*San Diego Union-Tribune*[80]

- "Study Links Breast Cancer, Hormone Use."—*Los Angeles Times*[81]
- "Maker of Fen-Phen Paid for Articles: Lawsuit Says Wyeth Hid Dangers Linked to Weight-Loss Drugs."—*Associated Press*[82]
- "Liver Toxicity with Prostate Cancer Drug Eulexin."—*Worst Pills, Best Pills News*[83]
- "Trovan Associated with Liver Injury and Death."—FDA[84]

Shocking? Knowing how the drug companies operate, it is no shock when new dangers are revealed with drugs we've been using for decades. It is no shock when:

- In 2000, the *Archives of Internal Medicine* reports that anti-inflammatory drugs have been linked with congestive heart disease.[85]
- In 1999, the *British Medical Journal (BMJ)* reported that SSRI antidepressants (e.g., Prozac, Zoloft, Paxil) have been linked with increased risks of gastrointestinal bleeding.[86]
- A 2000 *Los Angeles Times* headline announced that frequently prescribed drugs for high blood pressure (beta blockers) have been linked with diabetes.[87]
- In 2000, the *Annals of Internal Medicine* reported that drugs relaxing the muscles of the lower esophagus have been linked with increased risks of esophageal cancer.[88]

Unfortunately, revelations like these aren't new. These and many more surfaced in each of the thirty years since I earned my medical degree.

Of course, these incidents represent only *reported* adverse effects—the tip of the iceberg. Consider digoxin, the best-selling heart drug. According to an article in *JAMA*, the FDA receives about eighty-two reports annually involving digoxin, yet "a systematic study of Medicare records disclose 202,211 hospitalizations for digoxin adverse effects in a seven-year period."[89] That's more than 28,000 reactions per year—of which the FDA receives eighty-two.

THE GREAT TRAGEDY of it all is that so many side effects are avoidable. Prozac, perhaps the most famous breakthrough drug since penicillin and insulin, serves as a perfect example. Prescribed 24,742,000 times in 1999, Prozac causes side effects in a large proportion of the people started on it. Sexual dysfunctions alone occur in 33 to 50 percent or more of Prozac users.[90–92] Plus, the drug has repeatedly been linked to incidents of psychosis, suicide, and violent behavior. I saw some of this myself. But when I began individualizing my use of Prozac to fit the needs and tolerances of patients, side effects dropped dramatically, and the percentage of my patients obtaining good responses far exceeded Eli Lilly and Company's own claims.

Pfizer developed Lipitor to be extremely powerful in lowering blood cholesterol levels, so that with aggressive marketing, Lipitor could surpass better established, more proven competitors. With 48,791,000 prescriptions filled in 2000, Lipitor has accomplished this, but it has also triggered more reports to me about side effects than the other five drugs in its class combined. Perhaps this is because the standard dosage of Lipitor is so strong; it is far stronger than many patients actually need or can tolerate.

Similar problems exist in the way drug companies research and market many other top-selling drugs today. There is no doubt that popular drugs such as Zocor, Vasotec, Norvasc, Viagra, Motrin, Voltaren, Premarin, Prozac, Lipitor, Celebrex, Zestril, Allegra, etc., are very effective—I want to emphasize this—but today's methods of producing and prescribing these drugs do not include minimizing their risks. Of course, pharmaceutical companies cannot study everything, but as subsequent chapters will show, current research is woefully deficient in anticipating and avoiding *foreseeable* problems—problems that could be avoided by producing and prescribing medications to fit people.

The drug companies reject the assertion that their medications are not safe. "Do unsafe drugs enter and remain in the marketplace? Absolutely not," stated Bert Spilker, a senior vice president for the Pharmaceutical Research and Manufacturers of America (PhRMA), according to the *Los Angeles Times*.[93]

The drug companies also claim that they need large earnings—$124,835,595,000 in 1999—to conduct their research. They have a point—to a point. Aggressive research is indeed essential. The medications produced by the pharmaceutical industry have greatly improved the quality and length of life of millions of people. But this justification loses credibility when:

- Just one of every five dollars the drug industry collects goes to drug research.
- Some drug companies spend almost twice as much money for marketing and advertising than for research.
- Drug industry profit-taking is so large it outstrips every other industry by far.[94]

As Dr. Angell stated in a second astonishing 2000 article in *The New England Journal of Medicine* ("The Pharmaceutical Industry: To Whom Is It Accountable?"): "An industry so important to public health and so heavily subsidized and protected by the government has social responsibilities that should not be totally overshadowed by its drive for profits. There needs to be a better balance between the interest of the shareholders and those of the public."[95] Indeed, and this balance should begin with improving drug research and development in order to ensure drug safety and to end the side-effect epidemic.

The sad irony is that not only would patients, physicians, insurers, and health-care organizations benefit from reducing the high incidence of medication side effects, but so would the drug companies. When 50 percent or more of patients quit treatment for conditions such as high blood pressure,[96,97] high cholesterol,[98,99] and osteoporosis,[100,101] no one wins. These patients become exposed to markedly increased risks of premature disease and death, and the health-care system is burdened with billions in extra costs. However, if the priority in producing medications wasn't expediency but maximizing the benefits while minimizing the risks of medication treatment, many of these problems could be avoided. And keeping patients satisfied and in treatment would increase drug sales.

JUST BECAUSE SIDE effects are all too common, this doesn't mean they must be. In a 1999 article in *JAMA*, Dr. Wood stated, "Drug safety will improve only when it is viewed as a cooperative venture between regulator, industry, and prescriber, when all parties are prepared to engage in open dialogue so they may learn from the past with a view toward improving the future."[102]

This dialogue should have begun long ago, because ending the side-effect epidemic doesn't require some new insight or discovery: It simply requires restoring sound, practical, scientific principles to the ways we research, develop, regulate, and prescribe medications. As *Over Dose* will demonstrate in detail, we already have all of the information we need to do this—*to drastically reduce the occurrence of medication side effects and to end the side-effect epidemic today.* We have so much information that, by using it in the manner I will describe in subsequent chapters, patients can have great influence on how medications are prescribed to them. In doing so, they can greatly increase their chances of a positive response to medication treatment while greatly reducing their risks.

The side effects Alex endured should never have occurred. Once they did occur, they should have been promptly curtailed. Alex's disorder should have been easily and quickly controlled. This book will explain how—and how other patients and their physicians can do the same with their medications.

Ten Medications Withdrawn from the Market Since 1997 Because of Serious, Often Lethal Side Effects

- **Rezulin.** Given fast-track approval by the FDA, Rezulin was linked to sixty-three confirmed deaths and probably hundreds more. "We have real trouble," an FDA physician wrote in 1997, just a few months after Rezulin's approval.[103] The drug wasn't withdrawn until 2000.
- **Lotronex.** Against concerns of one of its own officers, the FDA approved Lotronex in February 2000. By the time it was withdrawn nine months later, the FDA had received reports of ninety-three hospitalizations, multiple emergency bowel surgeries, and five deaths.[104]
- **Propulsid.** A top-selling drug for many years, the drug was linked to hundreds of cases of heart arrhythmias and one hundred deaths.
- **Redux.** Taken by millions for weight loss after its approval in April 1996, Redux was soon linked to heart valve damage and a disabling, often lethal pulmonary disorder. Withdrawn in September 1997.
- **Pondimin.** A component of Fen-Phen, the diet fad drug. Approved in 1973, Pondimin's link to heart valve damage and a lethal pulmonary disorder wasn't recognized until shortly before its withdrawal in 1997.
- **Duract.** The painkiller was withdrawn when it was linked to severe, sometimes fatal liver failure.
- **Seldane.** America's and the world's top-selling antihistamine for a decade, it took the FDA five years to recognize that Seldane was causing cardiac arrhythmias, blackouts, hospitalizations, and deaths—and another eight years to withdraw it.
- **Hismanal.** Approved in 1988 and soon known to cause cardiac arrhythmias, the drug was finally withdrawn in 1999.
- **Posicor.** For treating hypertension, the drug was linked to life-threatening drug interactions and more than a hundred deaths. An expert on the advisory committee said, "Posicor should not have been approved."[105]
- **Raxar.** Linked to cardiac toxicities and deaths.

Chapter 2

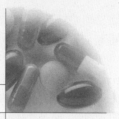

How Drug-Company
Policies Harm People

ONE OF THE FIRST principles of medical science is that when people are given the same dose of the same drug, their responses vary greatly. This is called *individual variation*. How much variation? According to the *AMA Drug Evaluations*,[1] individual variation with any drug can range from four- to forty-fold. That's a 400-to-4,000 percent difference in the dosage that may be required between one person and another.

We see this variation every day. Individual variation is why some people can handle a pot of coffee, and others can't handle a cup. It is why some people can drain a bottle of wine without a problem, while others can't handle a glass. Individual variation is also seen with every medication, prescription and nonprescription. Individual variation is why some people need 80 mg of Prozac or Lipitor, while others need only 2.5 mg of these same drugs, and the majority of people need doses somewhere in between.

The very wide range of individual variation is why *Goth's Medical Pharmacology*, a medical-school textbook for decades, states, "Many adverse reactions probably arise from failure to tailor the dosage of drugs to widely different individual needs."[2] And *Goodman and Gilman's The Pharmacological Basis of Therapeutics,* perhaps medicine's most respected reference, adds, "Therapists of every type have long recognized that individual patients show wide variability in response to the same drug or treatment method."[3] And Martin's *Hazards of Medication* warns succinctly, "The ultimate hazard is variability of patient response."[4]

Such variation isn't the exception: It is the rule. This is an everyday fact of medical practice, as I saw myself during twenty years of treating patients, and as scores of physicians, nurses, and pharmacists have reaffirmed to me.

The importance of matching the dose of a medication to the individual is obvious. It makes medical sense and common sense. So how would you feel if you took a medication but the side effects made you feel awful, and then you learned that the dosage the drug company recommended and your doctor prescribed was 100 to 300 percent greater than you really needed? And that with a lower, more individualized dose—a lower dose proven effective *in the drug company's own early research*—you probably would have avoided these side effects entirely? Yes, this really happens. Frequently. With dozens of top-selling medications. Here's one example.

Ella was 35 when diagnosed with rheumatoid arthritis in 1994. For the unrelenting pain, her doctor prescribed an anti-inflammatory drug, but the drug caused side effects Ella couldn't tolerate. So he prescribed another. Again, intolerable side effects. He prescribed another. More side effects. Finally, Ella's doctor prescribed Voltaren, which sometimes works when Motrin, Naprosyn, and others cause problems. That's why, for many years, Voltaren was the world's best-selling anti-inflammatory drug, and today Voltaren's generic counterpart, diclofenac, remains a top-seller. What dosage of Voltaren did Ella receive? Fifty mg three times a day, just as the drug manufacturer recommended. The first 50-mg pill sent Ella into a tailspin. Years later, the memory remained vivid.

"I felt wired, as if all of my muscles were quivering, like bugs crawling around inside. It was a terrible feeling, like I was going out of my skin." The reaction kept Ella awake all night.

The doctor switched her to another anti-inflammatory drug, then another. Switching patients from medication to medication is the standard approach. Why doesn't it occur to more doctors that the patient might simply need a lower dosage? Because the pharmaceutical industry is the dominant provider of drug information. Yet as I have demonstrated in several published articles, drug companies frequently do not provide information that shows that lower doses work.[5–8]

So when a patient develops a side effect, rather than simply reducing the dose without any extra cost to anyone, doctors do what they know best—write another prescription. One pharmacist described it perfectly: "If a medication doesn't work or causes side effects, most physicians just switch from one to another, then another, then another, until they either find a drug that works, or they or the patient give up. Very few physicians go to the trouble of adjusting drug dosages to fit their patients. Most don't deviate from the drug companies' recommendations. They don't individualize."

Medical schools teach doctors about the general principle of individual variation, but they don't teach how this applies to specific medications. It is assumed that when students begin seeing patients in later years, they will be taught how to individualize doses, but this usually doesn't happen. Young doctors learn from older doctors, who have little knowledge about lower, safer doses. And, of course, the most used drug reference among physicians is the *Physicians' Desk Reference (PDR),* which is supported by the drug companies, and which provides drug-company doses while lacking many lower, safer, effective doses that work.[9–12]

At least Ella's doctor cared enough to keep trying to help her in the only manner he knew. Still doubting her unusual experience with Voltaren, the doctor encouraged her to try it again. Ella's reaction was exactly as before. The doctor couldn't understand it. He had prescribed the medication exactly as recommended—not a milligram more. I sympathize with his predicament. Like most doctors, he wasn't trained to question the manufacturer-recommended doses of drugs. He was never told that the *PDR* contains only the information that manufacturers, with FDA consent, choose to provide, and that valuable low-dose data is frequently omitted. So it didn't occur to him to prescribe Voltaren at a lower dose, even though a smaller, 25-mg pill was available.

Voltaren's manufacturer, now called Novartis, didn't help. Before the company obtained the FDA's approval of Voltaren at the starting dose of 50 mg three times a day for rheumatoid arthritis (and for menstrual pain; for osteoarthritis, the dose is 50 mg twice daily), at least seven reports had been published demonstrating the effectiveness of Voltaren at 25 mg three times a day. That's 50 percent less medication. These studies were published in the *American Journal of Medicine,*[13] *Current Therapeutic Research,*[14] *Rheumatology and Rehabilitation,*[15] *Seminars in Arthritis and Rheumatism,*[16] *Journal of International Medical Research,*[17] and the *Scandinavian Journal of Rheumatology.*[18,19] The studies found that 25 mg three times a day of Voltaren was not only highly effective but also safer. One plainly stated: "In the trials in which we compared the 75 mg and 100 mg doses of diclofenac [Voltaren], in no trial did we show a significant difference between the two doses. One would expect, however, that with higher doses there would be some tendency for more unwanted effects . . ."[20]

Despite these findings, Voltaren was developed and FDA-approved at the standard higher dose, while the package insert, PDR write-up, and other drug company information omitted any mention of the low-dose studies. So Ella's doctor had no way of knowing that 25 mg three times a day of Voltaren worked, and that this low dose was not only easier to tolerate, but effective even for a tough disorder like rheumatoid arthritis. Like most doctors, *he assumed that if the manufacturer didn't recommend it, a lower dose of Voltaren wasn't effective. This is an inaccurate assumption that thousands of doctors make every day.*

But how can doctors even consider prescribing lower, safer doses if drug companies don't provide the data? It would be equally unwise to just guess at a dose. Inadequate treatment can cause harm too. That's why the information on lower doses is so important—and why its omission by the drug companies is a major factor in the side-effect epidemic.

Ella finally got fed up with the side effects and quit treatment. Today there is still no mention in Voltaren's 2000 package insert or *PDR* write-up about any of the studies with the 25-mg dose for arthritis.

WHY DIDN'T NOVARTIS recommend the 25-mg dose? Why didn't it at least inform doctors (and consumers, many of whom read package inserts or the *PDR*) about the effectiveness of this lower, safer dose? *Because the goals of drug companies often aren't the same as patients' goals.*

But aren't pharmaceutical companies concerned about medication side effects? Of course—to a point. A drug company doesn't want a new drug to cause any more side effects than necessary. On the other hand, getting a drug to the market quickly, before its competitors, is often worth billions and proves far more important to drug companies than determining the very best and safest doses for patients.

Besides, who are the main clients of drug companies? Who determines if a new drug will make billions? Not patients. Although it's your money and your body, you don't determine the drug's sales. Doctors are the arbiters of the fates of new drugs. In order for a drug to be successful, doctors must write the millions of prescriptions ordering it. If doctors aren't impressed, the drug fails, no matter its merits medically.

Doctors are the main clients of drug companies, not patients.

Therefore, drug companies tailor their medications to the needs and preferences of doctors. Whereas patients' first concern about medications is safety, drug companies emphasize other attributes to gain physicians' favor—and, in doing so, exacerbate the side-effect epidemic.

First and foremost, drug companies emphasize effectiveness. A new drug must be not merely effective, it must outclass its established competitors in order to get doctors to switch to it. Doctors do not switch to new, unproven, and unfamiliar drugs from the ones with which they already have extensive experience and confidence unless there is a compelling reason. The promise of superior effectiveness is compelling. As a 2000 article in *Primary Psychiatry* put it, "Physicians generally want to see a relative advantage of the new treatment over the one it will replace."[21]

What produces maximal effectiveness? Higher doses. With most medications, effectiveness—and side effects—increases with increasing doses until toxicity is reached. So, when drug companies recommend higher doses of prescription drugs, they are also increasing the risks of side effects.

For example, Lipitor is the top-selling drug for treating high cholesterol and, prescribed 48,791,000 times in 2000, the second bestselling drug overall. Lipitor is marketed at a very strong initial dose, the most powerful initial dose in lowering cholesterol of all of the drugs of its group. Thus, Pfizer Inc can impress doctors and patients that the initial dose of Lipitor reduces cholesterol to preferred levels better than any other drug. This claim is used extensively in Lipitor's advertising, and it has been instrumental in Lipitor's surpassing well-established, better-proven competitors such as Zocor and Pravachol.

The catch is that most side effects with these drugs are dose-related. The more potent the dosage, the greater the risk of side effects. Moreover, although patients will take Lipitor for decades, we have no idea whether unforeseen, long-term side effects may occur— and potential long-term side effects will likely be dose-related. So while Pfizer boasts that Lipitor is so strong that doctors only have to prescribe the initial dosage to most patients, it doesn't mention that this dosage is 100 to 400 percent greater than millions of patients need.

I have been contacted by patients who have had awful reactions to Pfizer's recommended initial dose of Lipitor. There are Web sites with hundreds upon hundreds of cases, some so severe that people are disabled. Many of these reactions might have been avoided by using lower, safer, proven-effective doses of Lipitor—doses that better fit these patients' needs and tolerances—but these doses are not even mentioned in Lipitor's package insert or *PDR* description.[22]

Producing and promoting drug doses that are unnecessarily high for millions of patients does not conform to fundamental medical principles. "To think that the same dose will do the same thing to all patients is absurd," Dr. Raymond Woosley, the chairman of the department of pharmacology at Georgetown University, stated in the *Drug Therapy* article "Is Standard Dosing to Blame for Adverse Drug Reactions?" He added, "Patients need to be titrated, starting with the lowest possible dose that could have the desired effect."[23]

In an October 1999 interview with *The New York Times,* Carl Peck, a former director of the FDA's Center for Drug Evaluation and Research, stated, "One dose fits all is a marketing myth, but it's the holy grail that every drug company tries to achieve."[24]

When Voltaren was introduced, it had to outperform Motrin, Naprosyn, and other well-established competitors. The effectiveness rates with 50 mg of Voltaren three times a day were more impressive than with 25 mg three times a day, even though the lower dose was quite effective and undeniably safer.

The medication marketplace is a very competitive world. At pharmaceutical companies, doctors usually don't make the final decisions—business people make them. In order to sell medications, good and bad, elaborate marketing and advertising strategies are necessary, and impressive rates of effectiveness are essential. "Pharmaceutical companies are waging aggressive campaigns to change prescribers' habits and to distinguish their products from competing ones, even when the products are virtually indistinguishable," wrote former FDA commissioner David Kessler. "Victory in these therapeutic-class wars can mean millions of dollars for a drug company. But for patients and providers it can mean misleading promotions, conflicts of interest, increased costs for health care, and ultimately, inappropriate prescribing."[25]

THE PROBLEM IS compounded by the FDA. The FDA employs a statistical method called an "intent to treat analysis," which requires drug companies to include all patients who quit treatment during the new drug trials—even patients who quit for reasons unrelated to the medication itself. The FDA's goal is to ensure the absolute effectiveness of the new drug.

However, this method forces drug companies to utilize unnecessarily high doses just to convince the FDA that the new drug works. In *Drug Therapy*, Dr. Woosley explained, "Drug companies use the highest possible dose just to account for those nonresponders who never even got the product." Gillian Woollett, an associate vice president for the Pharmaceutical Research & Manufacturers of America, added, "It's the regulatory [FDA] requirement to demonstrate efficacy that drives higher doses."[26]

But the drug companies are not innocent participants in this process. The FDA does not bar drug companies from researching and producing lower doses. Nor does it force them to omit important low-dose data from their product information. Indeed, some drug companies provide this data. For example, Merck recommends Zocor, its top-selling drug for lowering cholesterol, at a starting dosage of 20 mg/day, but the Zocor package insert also contains information about the effectiveness of 10- and 5-mg doses of Zocor, and Merck produces Zocor in these lower sizes. Unfortunately, many companies do not follow Merck's lead. They do not make their low-dose data readily available to doctors and patients, and they do not produce low-dose pills. In fact, in 1996, eight years after Voltaren was introduced, the manufacturer reduced the recommended initial dose for rheumatoid arthritis to 50 mg twice daily, but this is still too much for people like Ella, and it still ignores a half-dozen low-dose studies.

Why don't drug companies inform doctors and patients about lower, effective, safer doses? For example, with Voltaren, why not let doctors and patients choose between low and standard doses? With this information, Ella's doctor would have known simply to reduce her dose.

Producing a range of effective doses is simple, but doing so runs counter to the second major marketing strategy that drug companies use to attract doctors to new drugs: *ease of usage*.

With Voltaren, starting everyone at the same doses is easy to remember and easy to prescribe. If everyone receives the same dose, then doctors don't have to take the time to evaluate each patient and to then decide who may do best at 25 or 50 mg. Doctors don't have to ask whether each patient, like Ella, has had previous problems with similar drugs, or whether they are generally sensitive to medications, and then have to wait while patients answer. In fact, today there's more pressure than ever on doctors to work fast. Doctors who take their time with patients not only may make less money, but some also get harassed by administrators or partners for not packing in more patients by keeping the interactions brief.

Easy-to-use, simplistic, often one-size-fits-all initial doses with scores of drugs solve the problem for doctors. Simplistic dosing works for drug companies too. Limited doses are quicker and easier to research, cheaper to produce, and easier to market, requiring fewer guidelines and fewer pill sizes.

"Salespeople do not want to sell drugs that have to be titrated or individualized," a medical expert who performs studies for drug companies told me. "I have had numerous experiences with marketing representatives in which they have almost demanded a single pill strength and a single dose for all patients."

But simplistic, easy-to-use, unnecessarily high doses don't work for patients. These methods expose people to unnecessary, avoidable risks. The result is an epidemic of millions of side effects and thousands of deaths each year.

IF VOLTAREN WERE the exception among anti-inflammatory drugs, perhaps it could be considered a solitary bad example. But Voltaren isn't the only anti-inflammatory drug that works at lower, safer doses, nor is it the only one with crucial data omitted. For twenty-five years, the best known anti-inflammatory drug worldwide has been Motrin (ibuprofen). Low doses of Motrin were studied for rheumatoid arthritis, the pain after childbirth, menstrual pain, and pain from dental surgery. These studies showed that doses one half and even one quarter those recommended by the Upjohn Company—that's 50 to 75 percent less medication—were effective.

These studies appeared in the *American Journal of Medicine*,[27] Cur-

rent Therapeutic Research,[28] *Annals of Rheumatic Disease*,[29] *Clinical Pharmacology and Therapeutics*,[30,31] *Rheumatology and Physical Medicine*,[32,33] and *Compendium of Continuing Education in Dentistry*,[34] and yet, most doctors don't know about them. There are hundreds of medical journals, and most physicians read only a few. Even well-known journals like *JAMA* and *The New England Journal of Medicine* are read by a minority of physicians. Therefore, if the information about lower, safer doses isn't contained in the drug's package insert or *PDR* description—and it wasn't for Motrin—most physicians never know about it. Furthermore, if important information is omitted from the *PDR*, it is usually omitted from the bookstore drug references used by consumers.

Now consider: Anti-inflammatory drugs cause a higher rate of serious and fatal side effects than any other medication group.[35,36] The FDA receives more reports about anti-inflammatory drugs than any other drug group.[37] For many years, more than 16,000 deaths and 70,000 hospitalizations have been linked annually to anti-inflammatory drugs.[38,39] The relationship of anti-inflammatory drugs with gastric irritation, ulcers, and severe or deadly hemorrhaging, is well known, and these reactions frequently occur without any prior warning or pain, sometimes after just one or a few doses. These adverse effects are dose-related. Therefore, every expert has emphasized the importance of using the very lowest dose needed by each person. But even when drug companies have known about the effectiveness of lower, safer doses of these drugs, they haven't passed the information on to doctors and patients. This practice leads to people getting overmedicated with doses that are higher than they need, which in turn increases the likelihood of serious side effects and deaths.

VOLTAREN BECAME AVAILABLE in 1982, and Motrin in 1974. Drug companies and the FDA claim that the methods of drug development are much better today. Are they? Consider the case of Celebrex (celecoxib), which, after its introduction in 1999, became the fastest-selling new drug in history, and then totaled more than $2 billion dollars in sales in 2000. Before Celebrex was even approved,

Searle did a large amount of direct and indirect advertising about Celebrex's superiority over older anti-inflammatory drugs like Motrin, Voltaren, Relafen, Orudis, and others. The claim was that Celebrex is better than the older drugs because it causes fewer gastrointestinal hemorrhages, hospitalizations, and deaths. It was no secret that newer, safer anti-inflammatory drugs were badly needed, and Celebrex and Vioxx (rofecoxib, by Merck) may indeed represent a better wave. These drugs are specifically designed to reduce inflammation anywhere in the body without causing bleeding in the stomach or intestines. *Theoretically,* Celebrex and Vioxx should be safer, but only the mass usage of these drugs over several years will tell.

Although doctors were already prescribing Celebrex and Vioxx in record numbers, not everyone was convinced. Dr. Sidney Wolfe of Ralph Nader's Public Citizen Health Research Group doesn't believe these new, extremely expensive drugs have been proven sufficiently superior to the older anti-inflammatories. He cautions his readers to wait awhile longer until we learn the full truth about Celebrex and Vioxx. I don't entirely agree, because Celebrex and Vioxx do seem to cause less gastric irritation and less risk of hemorrhaging, ulcers, and death than older anti-inflammatory drugs. But I do agree that caution is warranted, for in the mid-1990's, a similar, supposedly new-generation anti-inflammatory drug, meloxicam, was approved in European countries, but it proved to be little better than older anti-inflammatory drugs and never appeared in the United States. In addition, Celebrex and Vioxx are associated with the same kidney damage, liver injury, nerve injury, depression, swelling, anxiety, hot flashes, ringing in the ears, increased sweating, elevated cholesterol, and other side effects of the older anti-inflammatories.

Will Celebrex and Vioxx ultimately prove safer than the older anti-inflammatory drugs? The real test is taking place right now, as millions of people of varying ages, sizes, states of health, and drug tolerances are prescribed Celebrex and Vioxx by their doctors. You are part of this experiment if you are taking Celebrex and Vioxx.

Because of the uncertainty about these drugs' safety, the FDA required the Celebrex and Vioxx package inserts to contain warnings about the possibility of gastrointestinal hemorrhaging. This proved to be a wise move: Within one month of Celebrex's approval, the FDA received ten reports of deaths and eleven reports of gastrointestinal bleeding related to Celebrex.[40]

For all of these reasons and more, experts emphasize the importance of using the very lowest effective dose of Celebrex and Vioxx. In fact, in the Celebrex package insert it says, "The lowest effective dose should be used for the shortest possible duration."[41] And: "The lowest dose of Celebrex should be sought for each patient." One problem: For Celebrex's most common usage (osteoarthritis, the arthritis from aging or trauma), Searle's recommended dose is one-size-fits-all. What is the point of telling people to use the "lowest dose" when the company recommends only one dose for everyone? This means that a 28-year-old, 250-pound linebacker, a 50-year-old, 100-pound woman, and a 90-year-old, 120-pound man who is taking five other medications will all receive the same dose for their osteoarthritis. Clearly the medication needs of these people are far from identical, but there is only one recommended dose for all of them.

A 13-year-old female gymnast will get the same dose too. Celebrex wasn't studied in children under 18, but it is inevitable that doctors will prescribe it to the young gymnast or a basketball prodigy or a football star with tendinitis, bursitis, or a strained back. Or your adolescent. Such usage is obvious: It should have been studied, but it wasn't.

The elderly don't get a lower dose of Celebrex, either, even though they should. Celebrex blood concentrations rise 50 percent higher in seniors *on average* (which means some seniors will get even higher blood concentrations) than in younger people. Not surprisingly, medication reactions occurred more frequently in older subjects in Searle's Celebrex studies.[42] Most of these side effects were dose-related. Yet, although osteoarthritis is most common in seniors, and drug metabolism is characteristically slower in this age group, they still receive the same dose of Celebrex as younger, heavier, and healthier adults. This is medically irrational.

The only group that receives a little dose flexibility with Celebrex is rheumatoid arthritis sufferers. They also are started at 100 mg twice daily, but if this isn't enough, doctors can bump their dose by 100 percent to 200 mg twice daily. This is a big increase that may be too much for many people. Two preset doses aren't enough flexibility for this widely differing population.

For all of these populations—adolescents, the elderly, as well as for many adults—a lower dosage of Celebrex would have been useful. And, in fact, a one-half dosage of 50 mg of Celebrex twice daily is significantly effective. This was proven in a 1999 study in the *Mayo Clinic Proceedings*.[43] Indeed, because the conditions of most of the patients in this study were rated as "poor or very poor," the study design actually favored higher doses of Celebrex. Still, the authors concluded, "Significant efficacy was also observed with the 50-mg [twice daily] dose of Celebrex compared with placebo." The lower dose also caused fewer patients to quit treatment because of side effects than Searle's recommended higher doses.

Interestingly, the authors made positive comparisons between Searle's recommended doses of Celebrex and the highest prescription dose of a popular, older anti-inflammatory drug, naproxen (Naprosyn). However, they failed to mention that if low-dose Celebrex worked for these severe cases, it would likely be highly effective for the millions of people with milder disorders. It would probably work well for people taking the lower prescription dose of naproxen—or taking over-the-counter naproxen (Aleve) or other anti-inflammatory drugs—while posing less risk of ulcers and hemorrhaging. Instead, the authors seemed to downplay the potential usefulness of low-dose Celebrex. Interestingly, the study was funded in part by Searle, which doesn't manufacture a 50-mg dose of Celebrex or mention low-dose Celebrex in its package insert or *PDR* description.[44]

Scientifically, there is no justification for failing to produce dosages that are safer yet effective or for failing to inform doctors and consumers about the lower, safer doses. Nor is there a justification for marketing Celebrex in only 100- and 200-mg capsules. Capsules can't be split, making it difficult for anyone to use a lower dose.

Voltaren, Motrin, and Celebrex would be just as profitable—even more so—by employing better methods that ensure safety and, by keeping side effects to a minimum, keep people in treatment. But how do you convince the pharmaceutical industry to expand its research and provide better-designed drugs when they are already reaping record profits? In more than half a century, we have seen no change in the policies of developing and marketing new drugs at unnecessarily high doses, of disregarding individual variation and making flexible dosing difficult, of designing doses to satisfy doctors' preferences for easy-to-use medications rather than for maximum safety, and of ignoring lower, safer, proven-effective doses.

In fact, these problems have worsened in the last decade. According to a March 2001 report in *Reuters Health*, "One in five drugs approved by the U.S. Food and Drug Administration ends up undergoing a change in recommended dosage after the drug hits the market."[45] Eighty percent of these changes were reductions—reductions that were prompted by side effects in patients after their physicians reported them to the FDA or drug companies. Only then were lower, safer doses considered—too late for the thousands or perhaps millions of patients already experiencing reactions. Moreover, drugs approved between 1995 and 1999 were twice as likely to require dosage adjustments than drugs approved previously.

These findings came from an analysis of Dr. James T. Cross, a medical officer at the FDA, and Dr. Carl C. Peck, a former director of the Center for Drug Evaluation and Research at the FDA. Dr. Peck has been writing for a decade about the deficiencies in the drug companies' research and the consequences of their failure to produce proper dosages for their new drugs. This new analysis underscores his point—and my point—that the initial doses of many new drugs are too high, and that they provoke many avoidable side effects in patients.

Lowering the recommended dosages of drugs years after their approval isn't a solution. Doctors don't reread the information about medications every time they prescribe them. Once doctors have learned the dosages of new drugs, that's what they use. This is why it is so important for drug companies to determine and produce the lowest effective medication doses from the outset, because changing the

34

doses later not only means that people have been harmed unnecessarily, but it also doesn't keep doctors from continuing to prescribe the original, unnecessarily high doses.

Furthermore, although some drug doses are eventually reduced, many that should be reduced aren't. Top-selling drugs like Voltaren, Motrin, Celebrex, and many others have been proven effective at lower, safer doses, but these are not the doses that drug companies continue to recommend to physicians or that physicians usually prescribe to patients.

Why Don't Drug Companies Produce Doses That Fit Individuals?

- **Cost.** Thorough dose research costs a little more, but it would save billions in health-care expenditures that side effects necessitate (extra doctor visits, extra prescriptions, lost work, avoidable hospitalizations, avoidable deaths). Yet, pharmaceutical companies don't pay for these expenditures, so there is no immediate financial incentive for undertaking better research.

- **Urgency.** Brief, limited dose studies help get a new drug onto the market ahead of its competitors. This is a top priority: Profits, bonuses, and jobs depend on it. Thus, drug companies are motivated to do as little as required, and that's exactly what many do.

- **Effective advertising.** Higher doses produce higher efficacy rates, which makes great advertising, even though these higher doses also produce higher side-effect rates. Simple dosing also makes good copy.

- **Pleasing doctors.** Easy-to-use dosing regimens save doctors' time. The less time spent with each patient translates into more patients per hour.

- **Weak FDA regulations.** The FDA's powers are limited in requiring the pharmaceutical industry to perform better research and provide vital low-dose information to physicians and patients.

- **No public pressure.** Public outrage about the side-effect epidemic is virtually nil. Patients usually blame doctors when dose-related side effects cause harm, not the drug companies that determined the dose. With few exceptions, pharmaceutical companies have rarely been held accountable.

- **Doing things right is risky.** Companies that might spend the extra money to improve research run the risk of being beaten by less-conscientious competitors. The urgency of market dynamics sometimes works against good science.

- **Basic economics.** With record profits and weak regulation, what incentive does the pharmaceutical industry have to change anything? Why invest more in better research that may decrease short-term profits and the value of drug-company stock and corporate executives' options?

How Drug-Company Policies Cause Problems for 50 to 75 Percent of Patients Taking Prozac

NO ONE EXPECTS business enterprises to act like charitable organizations. However, we do expect companies to draw the line when their policies cause harm. Unfortunately, for decades the pharmaceutical industry has failed to avoid causing unnecessary harm because its policies have been designed to maximize marketing strategies and sales rather than consumer safety. Prozac, which was taken by 38 million people worldwide between 1988 and 2000, and for which American doctors wrote 24,742,000 prescriptions in 1999 alone, offers a striking example.

Prozac is one of the true breakthrough drugs of the twentieth century and the number-three top-selling drug in America at the start of the twenty-first century. It is a very effective medication. But the antidepressant also causes millions of side effects that could easily be avoided. But they aren't, mainly because of how Prozac's manufacturer, Eli Lilly and Company, developed the drug and how doctors prescribe it.

Prozac became available in late 1988. The drug seemed very promising, but based on my long experience prescribing antidepressant medications, Prozac's one-size-fits-all starting dose of 20 mg worried me. I knew this couldn't be right. Years of experience as a medication expert had taught me that different people responded very differently to drugs, and that if I didn't tailor the dose accordingly, especially the initial dose, side effects would frequently occur.

Experience had taught me to heed the differences in people's ages and sizes, and to ask about previous medication reactions and about sensitivities to coffee or alcohol. People with such sensitivities often developed side effects to standard, manufacturer-recommended doses of powerful drugs like Prozac. Typically, I started these people at low doses, but with Prozac this was difficult because Prozac was produced in only one size, a 20-mg capsule. It didn't matter if you were small, old, frail, or took a dozen other medications—even if medically you had an excellent reason to start with a low dose of Prozac—still Lilly recommended 20 mg/day initially.

By the time I prescribed Prozac at Lilly's recommended dose to ten people, I knew there was a problem. Half of them did extremely well. Prozac was clearly a breakthrough drug. But the other half experienced side effects, and many weren't mild. Jean G. became so nervous and agitated with her first dose of Prozac, she couldn't work. It took two days for her body to calm down. Laura S. developed full-blown panic attacks with a racing, pounding heart, severe anxiety, trembling, profuse sweating, hyperventilation, and inability to concentrate or function. She'd never had a panic attack before and, after stopping Prozac, never had one again.

My worst case, though, occurred with Carol W.

Carol was 32 and only mildly depressed, so I didn't expect her to need much medication. After she'd taken the standard initial dose (20 mg) of Prozac for a few days, I received a frantic call from Carol's husband, Bob. Carol had felt increasingly disoriented and confused. Now she was psychotic, her mind spiraling out of control. Carol knew she was in trouble but refused to go to a hospital. Bob agreed to stay home, hold Carol's hand, feed her, and lead her to the bathroom. I spoke with Carol and Bob hourly, prescribed a mild sedative to calm

her down, and we all waited. Fortunately, Carol remained cooperative. Twenty-four hours later, she was greatly improved. After another
day, she was nearly back to normal. I breathed a sigh of relief. It was
the most severe drug reaction I encountered in my twenty-plus years
of clinical medicine.

I wasn't the only one who encountered such severe side effects at
Prozac's lowest recommended dose. A colleague had a patient who
became so agitated from Prozac, she wanted to ram her car into a wall.
She resisted the impulse, the doctor stopped the Prozac, and the agitation and impulse disappeared.

Then, just after Carol's incident, the media began reporting stories
about impulsive suicides and violent behavior by people taking
Prozac. Lilly insisted Prozac was safe. Congressional hearings were
held. I couldn't help being reminded of Carol's reaction. It would
have been a disaster if she hadn't been a stable person. Or if her husband hadn't been supportive. Or if her reaction occurred while she
was driving, or at work, or alone with her children. That's probably
what did happen to those who made headlines. Carol was a stable person, but that's not true of everyone who is prescribed Prozac. Some of
the casualties probably had no support, or were filled with hostility or
self-hate. Or maybe some were simply even more sensitive to Prozac
than Carol was.

I BEGAN HAVING patients open the Prozac capsule and mix the
powder in juice, then take one quarter or one half of the liquid each
day, thereby getting doses of 5 or 10 mg. This not only prevented a lot
of side effects but greatly increased the success rate. A few other doctors did the same thing, but most didn't. Most still don't use low-dose
Prozac, even in appropriate cases, even though lower-dose pills are
now available. I still receive letters and calls from people being overmedicated at the standard doses—that is, Lilly's doses—of Prozac.

I discussed my patients' reactions with a Lilly representative. He
insisted that the dosage couldn't be the problem. The drug company's research had been thorough. I wasn't reassured, so one day
I left the office early and went to the medical library to see if any

doctors had reported similar difficulties with Prozac. There I discovered a study that ultimately led me to examine the entire side-effect problem.

The study was published in *Psychopharmacology Bulletin* in March 1988, *before* Prozac was approved by the FDA.[1] It raised serious questions about the 20-mg dose. In this study, a dose of only 5 mg, 75 percent less medication, nearly equaled the 20-mg dose in its effectiveness. The 5-mg dose helped 54 percent of patients, while the 20-mg dose helped 64 percent. In other words, increasing the dose 400 percent, from 5 mg to 20 mg, helped just 10 percent more patients. And, not surprisingly, the larger 20-mg dose provoked more side effects and forced more patients to quit treatment. The authors suggested more studies to confirm the good results with the 5-mg dose, but Lilly proceeded with its application for the FDA's approval of Prozac—with 20 mg as the starting dose for everyone.

For many decades we have known that the dose is the key factor in the occurrence of most side effects. In 1978 *Hazards of Medications* stated, "Always administer the smallest amount of the least potent drug that will achieve the desired therapeutic effect."[2] Other drug references universally agree. Yet, it wasn't until the landmark study in *JAMA* in 1998 that the medical community realized how key the dosage is in preventing or causing side effects.

In addition to revealing that more than 100,000 deaths and 2,000,000 severe side effects occur from medications in U.S. hospitals annually, this study was designed to identify the origins of these side effects. To do this, the authors excluded other causes of medication problems, such as errors by physicians or pharmacists, and limited their attention to side effects caused directly by the medications themselves. The study showed *"that there are a large number of serious adverse drug reactions even when the drugs are properly prescribed and administered."*[3] Fully 76.2 percent of the side effects tallied in the *JAMA* study were dose-related, meaning that the problem wasn't the drugs themselves but the drug-company-recommended doses, which are just too strong for too many people.

This finding agreed with an earlier study that found that of all the reports of medication reactions submitted to the FDA in one year, 71 percent "involved toxic reactions to usual doses of drugs."[4] Moreover, even reactions that we do not usually consider dose-related—reactions such as allergic phenomena and drug interactions—are worse and more frequent at unnecessarily high doses. Many of these reactions would not occur at all if medication doses were properly matched to people.

However, the FDA made no objection to the one-size-fits-all initial dose of 20 mg, nor did it require Lilly to conduct further studies on the lower, safer 5-mg dose. It didn't even require any mention of this lower dose in Prozac's package insert or the *PDR*, which would have at least warned doctors about the sensitivity of some people to Prozac and provided them with an explanation when their patients reacted adversely. Instead, neither doctors nor patients were informed about low-dose Prozac, and they still aren't informed by the Prozac package insert or *PDR* description.

Now I understood why so many of my patients reacted adversely to Prozac. They were getting overmedicated. They were getting doses 100 to 400 percent greater than some of them needed. It wasn't just my patients: In one study, 39 percent of patients quit taking Prozac because of side effects.[5] This is a dreadful rate, but perfectly believable from what I saw.

I DIDN'T PRESCRIBE low-dose Prozac to everyone. I tailored the dose to the individual. For example, if the person was small, elderly, or physically ill, or had a history of side effects or sensitivities to drugs, I started Prozac at 5 or 10 mg/day. Often this was all that was needed. In several cases, just 2.5 mg was required.

If the person was experiencing a mild type of depression, I also started lower. This issue isn't explained in the dosage guidelines of the Prozac package insert or *PDR* description, or in many other professional or consumer medication references, so it is usually overlooked by doctors, but Lilly's recommended doses for Prozac were determined in patients with major depression, a severe disorder. Milder disorders occur more commonly than major depression, and among my patients milder disorders usually responded to milder doses of Prozac. This is a common occurrence with many types of disorders and drugs.

Many people didn't have a history of medication sensitivities but wanted to begin cautiously, so we agreed to start low too. When this worked, we avoided higher doses that might have caused side effects. When it didn't, we simply upped the dose—but more gradually than the 20–40–60-mg protocol recommended by Lilly. It was the patients' choice, as it should be. Patients are entitled to informed consent, which means informing them about dosage choices and giving them some say.

Some people knew from experience that they usually required full doses and experienced few side effects, so I started them at the standard 20-mg dose. Most did fine, but a few got side effects that required lowering the dose after all. Others required higher doses. The standard approach is to increase by 20 mg at a time: a 20–40–60–80-mg strategy. But these jumps were too large for some patients, and increasing from 20 to 40 mg or from 40 to 60 mg provoked side effects. So instead of following the usual protocol, I often increased people from 20 to 30 mg or from 40 to 50 mg. This worked very well, avoided side effects, and kept the daily dosage to a minimum.

The goal was to fit the Prozac to the person, not the person to Prozac's doses as chosen by Lilly. By fitting the dose to the person, far fewer problems occurred. The rate of Prozac side effects among my patients dropped dramatically. My success rate climbed to around 80 to 90 percent, far exceeding Lilly's results. Clearly, the problems with Prozac weren't due to the drug itself, but to the doses recommended by Lilly and prescribed by physicians.

MEANWHILE, THE CONGRESSIONAL hearings on Prozac commenced. I wasn't surprised when the findings were inconclusive, because there was no way to prove that Prozac was causing suicidal and homicidal reactions; these reactions occurred too infrequently to establish a clear statistical trend. But this didn't mean that Prozac hadn't played a role.

I was surprised by one thing: Through all of the hearings, no one raised the issue of the Prozac dose. No one questioned the fact that the violent reactions were caused by doses that were simply too strong for some people, just as Carol had experienced. Yet, when drunk drivers kill other people, it is standard procedure to measure their blood levels and find out how much they drank. We understand that alcohol's dangers are dose-related. But no one applied this same simple logic to the Prozac reactions.

CONCERNED ABOUT ALL of these things, I began researching other drugs and found similar problems. To my surprise, these problems didn't involve just a few drugs, but many drugs. Virtually all of Prozac's competitors, including top-sellers Zoloft, Paxil, Luvox, Serzone, Effexor, Wellbutrin, Elavil, Tofranil, Pamelor, and Norpramin, can be used in lower doses. But the problem didn't stop with antidepressants; it extended to all groups and types of medications. That's when I realized that many of the millions of side effects annually—the side-effect epidemic—were preventable. As experience had taught me with many medications but most vividly with Prozac, if medications are developed properly by drug manufacturers and prescribed properly by doctors, many side effects can be avoided.

Doctors assume that the doses drug companies recommend are carefully chosen to avoid side effects as much as possible. That's what I had assumed. That assumption is dead wrong.

Meanwhile, other researchers began studying Prozac at lower, safer doses—10 mg, 5 mg, and even 2.5 mg, depending on the disorder. Articles about lower doses appeared in *The New England Journal of Medicine*,[6] *Journal of Clinical Psychopharmacology*,[7] *Conn's Current Therapy*,[8] *The American Journal of Psychotherapy*,[9] and repeatedly in the *Journal of Clinical Psychiatry*.[10–13] Despite this convincing data, however, the vast majority of doctors continued to start patients at 20 mg of Prozac. They still do. The result? A rate of side effects that continues to be excessive. In Lilly's own studies, patients taking Prozac reported:[14]

- insomnia in 28 percent of Prozac users
- anxiety-nervousness in 28 percent

- nausea in 26 percent
- headaches in 21 percent
- sexual dysfunctions in 18 percent
- sedation in 17 percent
- low energy in 15 percent
- dry mouth in 12 percent
- stomach pain in 10 percent
- tremor in 9 percent
- profuse sweating in 7 percent

Add these numbers and it amounts to 191 side effects per 100 people! And these are just the most frequent side effects. Lilly lists scores more, nearly all of them dose-related. At lower doses, they would either not occur at all or at least be milder.

So why didn't Lilly develop lower doses to reduce these high rates? To be successful, Prozac had to outperform Elavil and Tofranil, its extremely well-established, highly successful competitors. Elavil and Tofranil had been reliable, top-selling drugs for decades, and doctors had already seen several "newer, better" antidepressants arrive and flop. It would take quite a promise of effectiveness to get doctors to switch to Prozac. Higher Prozac doses provided higher rates of effectiveness with which to impress doctors in Prozac's advertising.

Producing Prozac with a one-size-fits-all initial dose would also be easier to market, because it would be easy and quick for doctors to use. Doctors wouldn't have to decide which patients required 5 or 10 mg: Everyone would get 20 mg/day. It would make Prozac quicker and cheaper to market, and more attractive and less complicated for doctors. Lower, safer doses of Prozac were not produced, and many of my patients and millions of others sustained potentially avoidable side effects.

THE SIDE-EFFECT rates listed above are only half of the story. It is hard to believe, but many of these rates are underestimates. Independent studies reveal substantially higher rates. A study in the *Journal of Clinical Psychiatry* reported that nearly 85 percent of people treated with Prozac complained of diarrhea, 70 percent had profuse sweating, and 32 percent got headaches.[15] In another, 22 to 34 percent of patients taking Prozac got insomnia that required another drug to control.[16] In seniors, 40 percent required sleep medication to control Prozac-induced insomnia.[17]

Weight gain occurs in 18 to 50 percent of people taking Prozac.[18] In one study, 25.5 percent of Prozac patients experienced weight gains of 7 percent or more.[19] An internist I know has gained thirty pounds since starting Prozac. Yet, this side effect is not widely recognized, and most doctors aren't even aware that people can gain weight on Prozac and deny the association when people complain. One researcher described the problem this way: "Some physicians tell patients, 'I can't understand why you're gaining weight—you're on an SSRI [selective serotonin reuptake inhibitor, e.g., Prozac, Zoloft, Paxil]."[20] Even when these side effects are recognized, many physicians overlook the fact that they can be minimized by simply using a lower dose.

In studies with Prozac, sexual dysfunctions—dose-related decreased libido, impaired orgasm or anorgasmia, impaired ejaculation, diminished sensation, impotence—have been reported in as many as 50 to 70 percent of Prozac users.[21–28] Practitioners have told me that they see sexual dysfunctions, which are dose-related side effects, in more than 50 percent of Prozac users. Indeed, delayed ejaculation occurs so frequently in men, sex therapists prescribe Prozac as a treatment for premature ejaculation. Yet, for many years Lilly maintained that sexual dysfunctions occurred in only a tiny percent. In the 1990 *PDR*, Lilly listed decreased libido at 1.6 percent, ejaculatory problems at 1.9 percent, and impotence at 1.7 percent, and many physicians relying upon these numbers dismissed the frequent complaints of patients. Now Lilly lists these overall sexual dysfunctions at 18 percent, still far below independent assessments. Physicians continue to underestimate the problem, and patients still tell me of doctors denying that Prozac may be causing sexual dysfunctions that began only after starting the drug. Other times, physicians tell patients that the sexual dysfunctions will diminish with longer exposure to Prozac, but this often isn't the case.[29]

In 1999, articles in the *British Medical Journal*[30] and *Primary Psychia-*

try[31] revealed that Prozac and similar antidepressants are associated with increased bleeding in the gastrointestinal tract, urinary system, and even the brain. These side effects are not frequent, but they are serious, and they are very likely dose-related. They also occur much more often in people who are also taking anti-inflammatory drugs. A 1998 article in *The New England Journal of Medicine* revealed that in contrast to what most doctors believe, Prozac and other newer antidepressants cause elderly people in nursing homes to fall almost as often as the old antidepressants they were designed to replace.[32]

The only protection against unforeseen side effects like these is to use the very lowest, safest dosage for each patient. We may not be able to anticipate which side effects will be discovered a decade after a drug is introduced, but we can certainly anticipate that new side effects will be uncovered. With Prozac and similar drugs, long-term side effects are being reported "far in excess of what was expected from clinical trial data," according to Dr. Norman Sussman, the director of psychopharmacology research at New York's Bellevue Hospital Center. "These observations contrast with what the clinical trials submitted to the Food and Drug Administration by pharmaceutical companies show."[33]

Whether dealing with side effects that are frequent or rare, mild or serious, immediate or long-term, with Prozac or any other drug, the best protection is to use the very lowest dosage that each patient actually requires, not a one-size-fits-all dosage. The essence of medicine is preventing illness, and preventing side effects necessitate using the lowest, safest drug doses.

NO MATTER WHICH statistics you use, the side-effect rates with Prozac are high—unnecessarily high, because the great majority of these side effects can be prevented or minimized with more careful dosing. This has been known for years. In 1995, Michael Wise, M.D., of the Department of Psychiatry at Louisiana State University stated what knowledgeable doctors have long recognized: "In my experience, not only does gradual titration produce as beneficial a therapeutic effect as starting with a higher dose, but it generally results in fewer side effects and a better rapport with the patient. In the end, efficacy is the same."[34] Today, such dosing is easily accomplished because Prozac comes in a liquid and a breakable 10-mg tablet, but few doctors prescribe either. Why? Because, except for the elderly or people with liver abnormalities, Lilly still recommends 20 mg or more as the starting dose for everyone beginning Prozac. Prozac's package insert and *PDR* write-up, which are written by Lilly, still don't contain a word about the effectiveness of 2.5, 5, or 10 mg of Prozac, so most doctors, 90 percent of whom rely on the *PDR* for dosage guidelines,[35,36] aren't aware of the possibilities. Neither are most of the 500,000 consumers who buy the *PDR* every year.

When you understand these problems, it is not surprising that twelve years after Prozac was approved, people were again raising the issue of Prozac-related psychoses, suicides, and violent acts. Recent books such as *Prozac Backlash*[37] and *The Antidepressant Era*[38] have made headlines by citing studies suggesting a connection between Prozac and such reactions. A May 2000 story at www.drkoop.com Health News began, "The question of whether Prozac, the most-prescribed antidepressant, can make some patients more likely to commit suicide just won't go away, despite repeated and categorical rebuttals by the drug's manufacturer, Eli Lilly and Co. Based on his experience as a suicide counselor and investigator, Dr. Ronald W. Maris, director of the Center for the Study of Suicide at the University of South Carolina, is firmly convinced that a risk exists."[39]

Since 1990, physicians have reported on non-suicidal patients who developed suicidal thinking on Prozac.[40–44] The reaction is not frequent, but with millions of people taking Prozac, even a small risk can result in large numbers. Dr. David Healy, director of the North Wales Department of Psychological Medicine at the University of Wales, contends that serotonin-enhancing antidepressants like Prozac have caused thousands of suicidal acts.[45]

In May 2001, a judge in Australia found that a high dose of another serotonin-enhancing antidepressant, Zoloft, was responsible for a 76-year-old man killing his wife of 50 years. "I am satisfied that but for the Zoloft he had taken," Justice Barry O'Keefe said, "he would not have strangled his wife."[46]

These reactions are believed to be the result of severe anxiety, agitation, or akathisia (an overwhelming physical and mental restlessness) that can become intolerable.[47] These types of symptoms are associated with antidepressants such as Prozac and Zoloft, as Alex described in the beginning of this book. And as with Alex and Carol, these reactions are typically dose-related.

Prozac isn't the only drug prescribed at doses that overmedicate people and provoke avoidable side effects. It is just one prominent example of an industry-wide problem. The flaws and shortcomings I've described in the research and usage of Prozac pervade the pharmaceutical industry and apply to many drugs. And, as with Prozac, most of these drugs' side effects are *dose-related*, meaning, that they are *preventable*. We don't need better drugs—we need better doses—doses designed to fit people.

Results of the "5-mg Study" Conducted Before Prozac Was Approved at an Initial Dose of 20 mg/Day for Everyone

In this study conducted before the FDA approved Prozac, 5 mg of Prozac produced a response rate nearly equal to doses 400 percent and 800 percent higher and caused fewer side effects. Yet Prozac was approved and marketed at a starting dose of 20 mg/day for everyone.

Prozac Dosage (mg per day)	Response Rate
5 mg	54%
20 mg	64%
40 mg	65%

Adapted from: Wernicke, J.F., Dunlop, S. R., Dornseif, B.E., Bosomworth, J.C., Humbert, M. "Low-dose fluoxetine therapy for depression." *Psychopharmacology Bulletin,* 1988, 24(1):183–188.

Early Comments About Low-Dose Prozac from the Medical Literature

- **The New England Journal of Medicine, 1994:** "The results of three dose-effect studies . . . [demonstrated that] a dose of 5 mg per day was as effective as any of the higher doses."[48]

- **Journal of Clinical Psychiatry, 1993:** "We conclude that starting fluoxetine at doses lower than 20 mg is a useful strategy because of the substantial fraction of patients who cannot tolerate a 20-mg dose but appear to benefit from lower doses. . . . Patients often benefitted clinically from treatment at lower doses, and failure to tolerate 20 mg/day of fluoxetine [Prozac] should not be taken as evidence that the agent cannot be used efficaciously in these patients."[49]

- **Conn's Current Therapy, 1993:** "Many patients respond to the starting dose of 20 mg per day, but a substantial proportion need lower doses (e.g., 2.5 to 10/day). . . ."[50]

- **Journal of Clinical Psychiatry, 1992:** Noting that the early studies on Prozac lasted just 4–6 weeks, during which time the doses were raised rather quickly, the author concluded: "Responses to fluoxetine [Prozac] are likely to be attributed to doses that are much above those required to achieve [a satisfactory] response." After reviewing other studies utilizing low-dose Prozac, he added: ". . . these data point to 5 mg/day as optimal, although there is no evidence that doses *below* 5 mg/day are not equally effective."[51]

- **Journal of Clinical Psychiatry, 1991:** "Today, it is clear, however, that the precept of pushing the depressed patient quickly to a high dosage of antidepressant medication is not the optimal strategy for serotonergic agents. 'Start low and stay low' may be the new watchword, particularly with . . . compounds such as fluoxetine [Prozac]."[52]

- **Journal of Clinical Psychiatry, 1991:** ". . . a suggested starting dose for treatment of panic disorder is often 5 to 10 mg/day of fluoxetine . . . patients with panic disorder are often quite sensitive to the drug."[53]

- **Journal of Clinical Psychopharmacology, 1987:** "Clinically, we have observed fluoxetine to be effective over a wide range with many patients requiring very low dosages. . . ."[54]

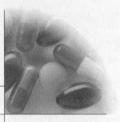

When New Drugs Are Approved, the Experiment Is Just Beginning, and You May Be Part of It: Viagra

ON MAY 29, 1998, Mike H. took Viagra. He was 65. He began to make love with his wife and passed out. Two days later he died. "I can't say that Viagra killed my husband, but I do say that Viagra contributed to it," his wife, Gerri, told *Newsweek*. "If I can make one man think twice before taking that pill, it's worth [speaking out]."[1]

Viagra represents both the best and worst of current medication treatment. To approve a new drug, the FDA must decide that it is "safe and effective," but these are relative terms. What the FDA really means is that statistically, in relation to millions of potential patients, the drug is *generally* safe, but not necessarily safe for everyone who takes it. As Robert Fenichel, M.D., a former deputy division director at FDA, has written, "Modern treatments can have beneficial effects . . . , but they can—and statistically will—do some harm too."[2]

When you take a medication for the first time, it's an entirely new experiment. Even if the drug company's research was thorough, there's still no way of knowing how the new drug will affect you. Drug studies establish trends and probabilities, but the range of individual variation is large and unpredictable. Each situation is, ultimately, unique. That's why many men have obtained excellent results with Viagra, others haven't, and others have suffered serious adverse reactions.

"My husband would never have taken Viagra if he had known there was any risk," Gerri told me. "His regular doctor sent him to a specialist just so he would get the best care, but the specialist hardly examined him and simply prescribed the standard dose. My husband was 65 with several medical problems and taking several other drugs, but he got the same dose as an 18-year-old. My husband's problem wasn't total: We did have sex on occasion without any problem. The first dose of Viagra, he died. We were close companions. My life will never be the same. I am not against Viagra—I'm against it being used so carelessly."

Does it make sense that a 65-year-old-man with several medical disorders and taking other medications should receive the same dose of any medication as a healthy 18-year-old? Of course not. Should the physician have considered a lower dosage for someone like Mike? Yes. Should there have been concerns about using Viagra in men with cardiac histories? Absolutely. But these weren't done. Dosing 65-year-olds the same as 18-year-olds isn't unusual today in the medical-pharmaceutical complex.

MIKE H. WASN'T the only Viagra casualty. First, 6 deaths were reported with Viagra, then 69,[3,4] then by November 1998, just seven and a half months after Viagra was introduced, the FDA reported 130 deaths in men taking Viagra. (Actually, a total of 242 deaths were reported, but the FDA excluded 112 deaths as unverifiable.[5])

"So many of them will say, 'I'm afraid to try it,'" William Catalona, chief of urology at Washington University School of Medicine in St. Louis, told *Newsweek*.[6] "I have some men [whose] wives have read or heard the stories about the fatal heart attacks and they just won't let them try it."

Who can blame them? Even considering that 3,000,000 men tried Viagra during its first eight months of availability, 242 Viagra-associated deaths (130 verified) are a lot—far more than the number of deaths linked with other drugs withdrawn by the FDA. Seldane, the top-selling antihistamine for over a decade, was linked with far fewer deaths—a dozen or so; yet, it was yanked in 1997. Rezulin, the new diabetes drug, was associated with about 60 deaths when the FDA finally gave it the hook.

Concerned about the Viagra reports, I spoke to several cardiologists about Viagra. Each of them felt that Viagra's impact on blood pressure could have had a direct role in many of these deaths. I awaited the next FDA report, but none was forthcoming, so I contacted the agency. I was told that the FDA had stopped analyzing the Viagra case reports and that no new summary report would be forthcoming. As of May 2001, thirty months after the last FDA report on Viagra, none has been published.

Others hadn't stopped counting. An independent analysis of Viagra's first thirteen months on the market, published in the *Journal of the American College of Cardiology*,[7] revealed *1,473 major drug reactions reported to the FDA, including 522 deaths, 517 heart attacks, 161 cardiac arrhythmias, and 119 strokes.* Of course, these numbers may be the tip of the iceberg, because, as explained in Chapter One, experts estimate that about only 1 to 5 percent of all serious medication reactions are reported to the FDA.[8,9]

SHOULD WE HAVE been surprised by these numbers? Not entirely. Just as with new models of cars and computers, errors are common with new drugs, which means unexpected side effects. Most often the side effects are unpleasant but not serious. Most often they are reversible. But sometimes they are serious and irreversible.

Melmon and Morrelli's Clinical Pharmacology states, "It would disappoint the patients and the profession to realize how truly little of the important medical consequences is known about a new drug at the time it becomes a salable product."[10] Even after sound early research, unexpected, serious side effects commonly occur when a new drug is introduced for general use. Premarketing research is conducted on several hundred to several thousand subjects, and people with other medical disorders or taking other medications are often excluded. Dr. Lon S. Schneider, professor of neurology, gerontology, and psychiatry at the University of Southern California, noted that drug company "trials may not generalize to typical patients, because they use highly rigorous subject selection or a dosing regimen that does not reflect how a medication is actually used in the community."[11] Thus, there is just no way to know how a new, powerful chemical is going to affect millions of patients of widely differing ages, genders, genetic make-ups, states of health, and innate sensitivities to medications, and using very different amounts of other medications or alcohol.

Indeed, unexpected side effects are so common that the first years after FDA approval are considered a distinct phase of drug research. The FDA even has a name for it: Phase 4. Phases 1 to 3 take place before FDA approval; Phase 4 takes place after. Yet, Phase 4 is the most important, most informative phase of drug research, for instead of being used in a few hundred or thousand carefully screened patients for a few weeks or months, the new drug is now used by millions of people of all types for years. Even when a manufacturer tries to cover the most likely possibilities, it can't cover them all, so that when the FDA approves a drug, there are many potential side effects and drug interactions that haven't been recognized. That's why Phase 4 usually reveals a lot more about how truly safe a new drug is in regular patients than all of the previous phases combined.

Knowledgeable doctors know this and use new drugs cautiously. Indeed, in a December 2000 article, Associated Press reporter Lauran Neergaard asked, "Should a savvy patient ever swallow a new medicine until it's been sold for a year? After all, that first year of sales often is when bad side effects are spotted." Dr. Raymond Woosley, a cardiologist and the director of the department of pharmacology at Georgetown University, answered, "I sure wouldn't. I don't personally, and I don't usually prescribe it unless I have to." Neergaard added, "Even the Food and Drug Administration's commissioner urges consumers to be cautious. It's advice Dr. Jane Henney says she'd follow herself."

Dr. Henney said, "Closely question when your doctor wants to switch to a brand-new remedy. Ask, 'How is this different? Why are you recommending this one over something I'm already taking?' If it's just because 'it's new and let's try it,' that's not a good enough reason."[12]

They aren't the only ones voicing these concerns. Dr. Brian Strom, an epidemiologist at the University of Pennsylvania, told the *Los Angeles Times* in March 2000, "It's important that people not rush out and want the newest drug." Commenting on the withdrawal of the diabetes drug Rezulin, he added, "The growing pressure on physicians to prescribe these drugs is driven by direct-to-consumer marketing. . . . We can't just rely on the FDA."[13]

But new drugs sometimes offer new or better solutions. Viagra is a perfect example. These drugs don't have to be avoided—they just have to be used with reasonable precautions. In fact, I felt so strongly about it that I published an article on the topic: "Should Patients Be Given a Low Test Dose of Viagra Initially?"[14] Of course they should, because: individual response to a new drug can never be predicted; Viagra has been linked with hundreds of deaths; low-dose Viagra works for some men; and, most of all, there's no hurry because erectile dysfunction isn't an emergency.

Unfortunately, reasonable precautions and common sense are often lacking with new drugs. "I am repeatedly dismayed when I see doctors prescribe new drugs without any hesitation," the chairman of a large department told me. "There's always extra risks with new drugs. There's always a shaking-out period when new side effects are frequently discovered. Yet, I see so many doctors who do not hesitate to prescribe brand-new drugs to patients, even when there are no advantages over other drugs that have been around for years and are just as effective. Of course, drug company sales reps spin their lines and provide handfuls of samples, but that's not reason enough—although apparently it is."

Viagra is a classic example: a very effective drug that has been directly linked with serious and lethal reactions, many of which might have been prevented simply by employing safer methods. Nearly all of the reported deaths linked to Viagra have been due to cardiovascular problems. Pfizer has maintained that Viagra has no direct cardiovascular effects, but in a letter to *The New England Journal of Medicine*, officers of the FDA challenged this claim and stated that in fact coronary artery activity "changed significantly from baseline values" following the use of Viagra. The officers added that because the studies of Viagra's effects on the cardiovascular system were so small, side effects that could occur in as many as 20 percent of Viagra users might have been missed. The officers concluded, "The inability to exclude side effects occurring in up to 20 percent of patients is not reassuring for a drug that is being used by thousands of men worldwide. Until much larger studies have been done, physicians and their patients should continue to exercise caution with regard to the potential for adverse cardiovascular effects of sildenafil [Viagra]."[15]

Some of the manufacturer's claims about Viagra's effects on blood pressure are also questionable. The package insert states that these effects are not dose-related,[16] but Viagra's effects on blood flow in the penis are obviously dose-related, and so are vascular side effects such as flushing and headaches.[17] In a review of eighteen studies, researchers found that the incidence of side effects, including vasodilation-related headaches, flushing, nasal congestion, and dizziness, "increased as the dose of sildenafil [Viagra] increased."[18]

Furthermore, there is evidence that Viagra's effects on blood pressure are indeed dose-related,[19] and it is likely that all of Viagra's effects on the circulatory system are dose-related too. This means that the serious cardiovascular reactions associated with Viagra might not have occurred or might certainly have been less severe if lower doses had been used. The fact that, within just thirteen months of Viagra's introduction, nearly fifteen hundred men have had heart attacks, strokes, or arrhythmias—or died—in association with Viagra suggests that Pfizer's recommended initial doses are too strong for some people. It's that simple.

Pfizer and the FDA have found many reasons for explaining Viagra-associated deaths. Many deaths have been blamed on people's age. But what age group did they expect would use Viagra—healthy teenagers? The average man with erectile dysfunction is over age 50.

Erectile dysfunction is by definition a disorder of older men. Viagra should have been designed specifically for the metabolisms and sensitivities of older men.

Some Viagra deaths have been blamed on sexual activity. But isn't Viagra designed to promote sexual activity? Without Viagra, these people wouldn't have been having sex. If these men were so unfit that enabling sex killed them, shouldn't their doctors have hesitated to prescribe Viagra or at least begun treatment in the safest manner possible? Moreover, some men dying with Viagra hadn't even begun to have sex.[20,21]

"The people who died had underlying cardiovascular problems," the *Los Angeles Times* quoted an FDA spokesperson.[22] But because of Viagra's known effects on the cardiovascular system, it should not have been a surprise that the drug might pose a risk for people with histories of heart disease, stroke, or other cardiovascular disorders. These people are well known to exhibit extreme sensitivity to drugs affecting blood pressure.

So why didn't Pfizer include adequate warnings for such people at the time Viagra was approved? Why didn't the FDA require it? According to Ralph Nader's *Public Citizen's Health Research Group,* men with some cardiac conditions were in fact excluded from Pfizer's Viagra studies. "The FDA cardiovascular advisory committee was completely bypassed during the six month approval process for Viagra," Dr. Sidney Wolfe stated. "This drug was dangerously rushed to the market."[23] Cardiovascular disease is a leading cause of erectile dysfunction, so it's obvious that men with heart disease would be among those trying Viagra. These men should have been among the most studied.

Finally in November 1998, after the death toll topped 242, the FDA required Pfizer to issue warnings about Viagra's use in people with cardiovascular disease, confirming what many critics believed was necessary from the beginning. The warning states that "serious cardiovascular events, including myocardial infarction, sudden cardiac death, ventricular arrythmia," as well as strokes and hypertension have been reported with Viagra usage.

After requiring these warnings, the FDA stopped actively monitoring Viagra-related deaths. Since November 1998, the FDA hasn't released any updated information. The agency hasn't even verified that the new warnings have had any impact. Yet, in May 1999, six months after the FDA's last report, a group of concerned cardiologists released its analysis of Viagra cases sent to the FDA.[24] The cardiologists tallied 522 Viagra-related deaths, revealing that more deaths had been reported per month after the new Viagra warnings than before. Still, no further data has been released by the FDA or Pfizer.

IF ALL THE serious reactions and deaths with Viagra are due to other factors, how do we explain reactions that have occurred in healthy people? Frank A., age 65, was visiting England with his wife. Before leaving the U.S., Frank got a prescription for Viagra. He took the first pill in England—and suffered a heart attack thirty minutes later.

Frank had no history of heart disease or any other contributing illness. He didn't even have a family history of heart attacks. He didn't smoke and drank modestly. He wasn't taking other medications. Nor could the heart attack be blamed on sexual activity. Frank and his wife hadn't even begun to have sex when the heart attack struck. In short, there was nothing in Frank's history or habits to explain his sudden heart attack except the Viagra. His doctors agreed and said so in the highly respected British journal *Lancet:* "Sildenafil [Viagra] should be considered as the most likely cause of his myocardial infarction."[25]

The FDA's absolving Viagra in every serious reaction and death defies credibility, especially when Viagra reactions have occurred in perfectly healthy men like Frank. In fact, most of the Viagra-associated deaths occurred in men with no risk factors. "No identifiable risk factor was reported in 67% of the patients who died," the *Journal of the American College of Cardiology* found.[26] Blaming Viagra reactions on factors such as mildly elevated blood pressure or cholesterol, cigarette smoking, or obesity also is questionable. That's why a cardiologist whose patient suffered a heart attack with Viagra told me, "I think the drug possesses real dangers. I think the FDA and drug companies are just sweeping it under the rug."

Pfizer and the FDA claim that Viagra has caused no more deaths than would be expected among several million men with the same medical problems (e.g., high blood pressure, heart disease, diabetes) commonly associated with erectile dysfunction and now engaging in sex. In other words, the association of these deaths with Viagra is coincidental: These men, undertaking sex, would have died anyway, with or without Viagra. I have never been convinced. As noted earlier, some Viagra deaths have occurred in men who didn't engage in sex. Others occurred in men whose erectile dysfunction was partial and who had repeatedly engaged in sexual activity without any problems before Viagra. To me, the explanations by Pfizer and the FDA weren't convincing, but was there any way to prove they were wrong?

Maybe so. Before Viagra, other medications were used to treat erectile dysfunction. They still are. Have these drugs been associated with a high incidence of heart attacks, strokes, and deaths? That's what you would expect if sexual activity and normal attrition in the population of men with erectile dysfunction are the culprits, because these drugs are used in the same way by the very same population of men as Viagra.

I obtained the FDA's adverse reaction reports involving Caverject, an injectable drug introduced in 1995 for treating erectile dysfunction, and I compared the frequency of deaths occurring with Caverject with the frequency occurring with Viagra.

Between 1998 and 1999, 407,000 prescriptions for Caverject were filled. In that time, three deaths were reported to the FDA. That's an incidence of one death per 135,700 prescriptions, or 7.4 deaths per million prescriptions of Caverject. How does this compare with Viagra? Using the FDA's statistics covering eight months in 1998, the incidence with Viagra was 1 death per 26,100 prescriptions (242 reported deaths per 6.3 million prescriptions), or 38.1 deaths per million. Comparing the numbers, Viagra was associated with more than five times the number of reported deaths than Caverject (38.1 vs. 7.4 deaths per million prescriptions). This difference is highly significant statistically.

I performed other analyses: The results were similar. As I reported in March 2001 in the *Annals of Pharmacotherapy*, Viagra-related deaths were being reported five to six times more frequently than deaths related to Caverject.[27] But maybe these statistics simply reflect that, because of Viagra's widespread publicity, doctors are alerting the FDA about Viagra deaths more reliably than about Caverject deaths. Undoubtedly this explains some of the difference, but I find it difficult to believe that if Caverject has been involved in the same frequency of deaths as Viagra, more deaths with Caverject wouldn't have been reported. After all, by mid-1998, doctors were well aware that any drug for erectile dysfunction might be associated with major side effects. Until proven otherwise, my analyses raise further concerns that Viagra may play a direct role in some deaths—and it is another reason for carefully matching the Viagra dosage to the individual.

ONE QUESTION I have been repeatedly asked: Should Viagra be withdrawn? That's another problem with our system: We go from denial to crisis, and then from crisis to overreaction, without ever taking the most rational step—simply fitting the dosages to people and thereby avoiding side effects.

No, Viagra shouldn't be withdrawn. Like Prozac, Voltaren, Celebrex, and just about every other drug I discuss in this book, Viagra is an excellent medication. The problem isn't the drug but how we are using it. Viagra is more effective and easier to use than any other treatment for erectile dysfunction. Seventy percent of the men who try Viagra get a good response. Without doubt, Viagra is a breakthrough drug. But if we used Viagra more scientifically, more carefully, especially when it was approved by the FDA and introduced for general usage, a lot of the risk, fear, uncertainty, and real dangers that have occurred with Viagra could have been avoided.

THE MOST IMPORTANT question about Viagra-related heart attacks and deaths is: What was the Viagra dosage? This is the key question, because many of Viagra's side effects, including its effects on the circulatory system, are dose-related. Yet, questions about dosage are rarely asked by doctors or patients. Even the media has missed the boat: They typically cover every aspect of a medication's dangers and provide quotes from experts, but rarely mention the dosage that caused the drug reactions. Few people, including physicians, seem to understand that whatever mechanisms underlie the problems with Viagra, Prozac, Voltaren, Motrin, Celebrex, and other drugs, the majority of all side effects are dose-related. In the landmark 1998 *JAMA* study, the authors found that 76.2 percent of all side effects were dose-related.[28]

Thus, despite the number of deaths associated with Viagra, I have not seen a single article or heard a single doctor or news reporter raise any questions about how Viagra is dosed. Both Mike and Frank took 50 mg of Viagra, the dose recommended by Pfizer for men ages 18 to 65. This is the same dose at which 78 percent of Viagra-related deaths have occurred. This statistic isn't surprising, because all men 18–65 aren't the same. There is a great difference in how an 18-year-old and a 65-year-old process medications. For example, liver and kidney function, so necessary for eliminating Viagra, drop 50 percent or more from age 18 to 65. The result is higher, longer, and more potent blood levels of Viagra in many older people.

Lumping such a large group together isn't medically rational. If you are 65, Pfizer recommends 50 mg of Viagra. If you are 66, Pfizer recommends 25 mg, a 50-percent lower dose, a huge difference pharmacologically. Does some dramatic bodily change occur between 65 and 66? Of course not. Someone 65 is more similar to someone 66 than someone 18, but the 65-year-old gets the same dose as the 18-year-old. Mike and Frank were 65, they were prescribed 50 mg of Viagra, just as the package insert recommended—just as it recommends for an 18-year-old.

Drug companies must, of course, provide guidelines for prescribing their drugs. But, as discussed in previous chapters, many drug guidelines are overly simplistic, gauged to make prescribing easy for doctors rather than to prevent side effects in patients. Mike and Frank might be fine if only they had been 66 instead of 65.

The drug companies' methods when releasing new drugs for general usage—for beginning the Phase 4 experiment—may explain many of the problems we are seeing. The way Viagra is dosed may also explain why the average age of men dying with Viagra is 64. My sense is that it's men 50 to 65 who are having most of the problems, because the 50-mg recommended dose may be too strong initially for some of them. Similarly, with Pfizer recommending 25 mg for all people 66 and older, this dosage may be too strong initially for men over 75 or 80, especially for those with other medical problems or taking other medications. However, Pfizer doesn't make a pill smaller than 25 mg and Viagra pills aren't scored, so starting with a lower dose for older men is difficult.

Pfizer does recommend adjusting the Viagra dose upward or downward according to the patient's response. In other words, if you are 18 to 65 and get a nasty side effect with 50 mg of Viagra, the doctor should then prescribe 25 mg. But not all Viagra-related reactions are reversible. Lethal reactions obviously cannot be reversed. Nor can heart attacks, strokes, and hemorrhages into eyes. Telling doctors to reduce a drug's dose after side effects occur is an ineffective, unnecessarily risky policy. Why not start lower and, once you know if Viagra is safe for you, have your doctor adjust the dose upward, if necessary, to your individual requirement?

Even the minor side effects that occur in 30 percent of Viagra users can ruin treatment. Severe flushing, headaches, stomach pain, heartburn, or visual distortions can be unpleasant and unnerving. John was eager to try Viagra and to no longer have to inject his penis with Caverject. John was 58 years old and, in accordance with Pfizer's recommendations, his doctor prescribed 50 mg of Viagra. John's first dose was his last.

"Your face gets very hot, you feel like your heart is beating faster than it should, there's anxiety," he reported in *Newsweek*.[29] He switched back to the injections. "I want to use something I'm comfortable with and I know is not going to kill me."

John's concern was understandable, but what he didn't know was that the side effects were dose-related. If he had started with a lower dose, John would likely have done fine. This is why Pfizer's strategy of reducing the dose after side effects occur is backwards. Experiences like John's and other men represent lost opportunities for men who could have benefited from Viagra if started at a lower dose, and they also represent lost opportunities for Pfizer, which loses long-term customers.

To avoid serious side effects, some experts have recommended giving men, especially men with heart problems, an exercise stress test before trying Viagra. This is a good idea, but it is no guarantee of safety. A recent case in *The New England Journal of Medicine* described a man whose exercise stress test was normal, but who two weeks later got a heart attack shortly after taking his first dose of Viagra.[30] With or without a stress test, it is impossible to predict how an individual will respond the first time taking Viagra or any drug. That's why experts have always advised starting with the lowest effective dose of any drug and then adjusting according to each person's response.

Starting with a low dose of a new drug—especially with a newly approved drug just entering Phase 4—isn't a new concept. Many drugs, particularly drugs affecting blood pressure, are intentionally started at low doses to identify people who are highly sensitive and reactive. In fact, this well-known medical phenomenon has a name: *first-dose reactivity*—the tendency of drugs to provoke reactions with their initial doses. This is a common phenomenon with many drugs. Case reports involving Viagra indicate that some of these reactions, like Mike's and Frank's, occurred with the first doses.

Because first-dose reactions and unforeseen reactions are inevitable, and because individual responses to drugs are highly variable and unpredictable, a basic principle of medication therapy is "Start low, go slow." "Start low, go slow" applies not only to Viagra but to most drugs. Starting with a low dosage allows a patient to put his or her toe into the water, so to speak, before jumping in blindly at the full medication dosage. This reduces the risk of severe reactions. Most conditions aren't acute. Treatment can be started gradually. Imagine how many lives might have been saved if Pfizer, the FDA, and physicians had merely considered this possibility.

Vital Information About Viagra That Was Lacking When Approved by the FDA

1. Inadequate information was provided on Viagra's effects on blood pressure at different doses and in different age groups.

2. Inadequate information was given on whether any patients in Pfizer's studies experienced dramatic drops in blood pressure with Viagra. This is the greatest concern with Viagra, but little information is provided.

3. Insufficient warnings were provided on the effects of Viagra on people with heart disease. This problem could have been anticipated, because erectile dysfunction commonly occurs in men with cardiac disease. It was only after the death reports began flowing in that the FDA required adequate warnings. If these warnings had been provided earlier, many lives would have been saved.

4. Inadequate studies were conducted on Viagra in combination with many drugs used for treating high blood pressure. Many men with impotence have hypertension and take antihypertensive drugs.

5. No studies or warnings were given about potential drug interactions with many drugs that may affect the body's ability to metabolize Viagra properly.

6. Insufficient Tagamet-Viagra information is provided. Pfizer mentions that Tagamet (cimetidine), a common heartburn and ulcer drug, increases Viagra's blood concentration by over 50 percent. But Pfizer doesn't suggest a lower initial Viagra dose for Tagamet users, who may have an increased risk of side effects.

7. Inadequate study and information was provided about the profound drug interactions with protease inhibitors (drugs for HIV and AIDS) and Viagra. Pfizer subsequently released new information, but questions remain.

8. Inadequate information is provided about Viagra and alcohol. Pfizer tells doctors it is safe in healthy people, but many men wth erectile dysfunction also have other disorders and take other medications. Is alcohol and Viagra safe for them?

64

9. Overly simplistic dosage recommendations fail to account for vast differences in drug response between individuals. This places many patients at unnecessary risk.

10. Unscored Viagra pills hinder flexible dosing. Pfizer seems very proud of its designer Viagra pill. But because Pfizer didn't score the pills for easy breakage, using half doses is difficult. This reduces the flexibility that doctors have in adjusting doses.

11. Inadequate, poorly defined precautions were given about the limits of what was known about Viagra when the FDA approved it. Gaps in information existed regarding Viagra with men with cardiac disease, with alcohol, with many antihypertensive drugs, with AIDS drugs, etc., but these were not clearly defined. Clear statements about the limits of Viagra studies are important so that doctors don't assume Viagra's safety in situations in which safety hadn't been assured.

Adapted from: Cohen, J.S. "Is the Product Information on Sildenafil (Viagra) Adequate to Facilitate Optimal Therapeutics and to Minimize Adverse Events?" *Annals of Pharmacotherapy,* March 2001, 35:337–42.

Why People Should Be Given a Low Test Dose of Viagra Initially

1. A low-dose test provides a scientifically sound, gradual approach that maximizes safety.

2. Low-dose testing avoids first-dose reactions and may help identify people unusually sensitive to Viagra's effects.

3. Test dosing reduces the risk of major adverse reactions and death. It also reduces the likelihood of minor side effects that frighten men or their partners and disrupt treatment.

4. Low-dose therapy may be sufficient for some patients.

5. Pfizer's dosage recommendations are simplistic and do not provide flexibility for the wide variation between patients in their responses to Viagra. Low-dose testing allows doctors and patients to fit the dosage to the individual.

6. Low-dose testing minimizes the risk of potential drug interactions. Many potential drug interactions with Viagra have not been studied.

7. Low-dose testing is safer for at-risk patients such as men taking other medications or having histories of unusual sensitivities to drugs.

8. Low-dose testing reduces the risks with untested uses of Viagra, such as in treating sexual dysfunctions caused by Prozac, Zoloft, Paxil, and other serotonin-enhancing antidepressants.

9. Low-dose testing allows patients to have a say in how Viagra treatment will be started. Patients should be involved in dosage decisions, because most side effects occur because of dosage problems.

10. Low-dose testing addresses the concerns that many people have about the safety of Viagra and may encourage them to get treatment.

11. Erectile dysfunction isn't an acute problem. It doesn't require immediate, intensive treatment. Most patients prefer safety to expediency.

Adapted from Cohen, J.S. "Should Patients Be Given a Low Test Dose of Viagra Initially?" *Drug Safety,* July 2000, 23:1–10.

Chapter 5

How Drug-
Company Policies
Harm Women

MEN HAVE SUFFERED the preponder-
ance of harm from Viagra, but over the years it is women who have suffered the brunt of inadequate drug-company policies.

Leslie was 32 when her doctor prescribed Relafen, a top-selling
anti-inflammatory drug, for her tennis elbow. The Relafen quickly
controlled her pain, but she began to get surges of anxiety. This was
unusual. Leslie had one of the coolest temperaments among the at-
torneys at her firm. Soon she was beset by a series of full-blown panic
episodes that made her a nervous wreck and disrupted her work.
Sleepless for a week from anxiety and a pounding heart, and facing a
pressure-filled new trial the next day, she went to an emergency room.

The doctor examined her and ordered blood tests and an electro-
cardiogram. Two hours later he returned and told Leslie there was
nothing wrong with her. Dismissing her objections, he gave her a prescription for Xanax, an anti-anxiety drug, and sent her home.

Leslie didn't believe she was okay. She didn't believe that her sudden, acute anxiety was "nothing." Just because the tests were negative didn't mean that a problem didn't exist. Nor did Leslie appreciate being brushed off as an overly emotional female. In fact, things had been going very well in her life. She was happily engaged and her law practice was thriving. Yet, she was now "climbing the walls," as she described it. The Xanax didn't help much, and Leslie didn't like relying on it. Tired and frustrated and getting nowhere, Leslie decided to stop all of her medications. Over the next forty-eight hours, her anxiety vanished.

Nervousness and insomnia are listed as side effects in the Relafen package insert and *PDR* description. The stated incidence of each is about 1 percent, but these may well be underestimates because anxiety is a common (and commonly overlooked) side effect of anti-inflammatory drugs, and the pre-marketing research on which these numbers are based often proves to be inaccurate (as I illustrated with Prozac-related sexual dysfunctions in Chapter Three). Even if the ER doctor didn't know this, he should have at least checked a drug reference. Unfortunately, his response isn't unusual. Doctors frequently dismiss or misdiagnose anxiety reactions. Even if they make the diagnosis, they underestimate how awful and disabling the symptoms can be and usually provide inadequate or inappropriate treatment, as this doctor did by prescribing Xanax, a drug that can cause dependency.

When you consider how SmithKline Beecham Pharmaceuticals markets Relafen, Leslie's reaction isn't surprising. SmithKline Beecham recommends a starting dose of 1,000 mg for everyone. Leslie weighs 103 pounds, and if 1,000 mg of Relafen is proper for a 200-pound man, it isn't difficult to conceive that this same dose may be excessive for a woman half this size. In fact, SmithKline Beecham states in the *PDR* that individual variation in response to Relafen is considerable, so dose-related side effects at the one-size-fits-all initial dose are almost assured in people more sensitive to Relafen than the norm—or people smaller than the "average" 170-pound person for whom drug companies design their doses. If Leslie had received a lower dose of

Relafen, her blood level of the drug wouldn't have climbed so high, and she probably would have avoided side effects that made her feel miserable, interfered with her work, and cost hundreds of dollars in additional medical expenses.

Leslie's reaction to Relafen could have been avoided or at least minimized if the drug company and ER doctor had considered that some people are more sensitive to medications than others, and these people are frequently small-framed women.

RELAFEN IS HARDLY the only drug with which women sustain avoidable side effects. The cardiac arrythmias and deaths that led to the FDA's 1997 withdrawal of Seldane, the top-selling antihistamine in the world from 1985 to 1995, primarily struck women. "Two-thirds of the cases were women," said Dr. Raymond Woosley in a May 1999 interview. Woosley has been a pioneer in the study of the differences of men's and women's responses to medications, but he wasn't entirely happy about his work with Seldane. "We missed it at first. It took awhile before it became clear. But then we realized this is too much to be a coincidence. There has to be a biologic basis for this."[1]

Woosley has seen similar arrythmias in women taking other medications. These arrythmias—potentially lethal irregular rhythms of the heart—are typically dose-related, the result of overmedication. This was the problem with Seldane: Some people couldn't handle the manufacturer-recommended dosage. In 1985, Marion Merrell Dow marketed Seldane at a one-size-fits-all 60 mg twice daily (i.e., 120 mg/day), but five years earlier a study published in the *Annals of Allergy* showed that 20 mg three times a day (i.e., 60 mg/day), one half the total daily dosage recommended by the manufacturer, was highly effective.[2] But the company never produced the lower dosage or even mentioned it in its product information, not even after Seldane's dose-related toxicity became known. So for eight years *after* Seldane's toxicity was revealed, doctors kept prescribing millions of prescriptions each year at the unnecessarily high manufacturer-recommended dosage, and people—the majority likely women—continued to sustain side effects.[3]

Woosley believes that as many as forty drugs available today can produce cardiac arrythmias, and with ten of these drugs women have a twofold greater risk than men. The reason for this difference isn't known, in part because little funding has been available to investigate it. For many years Woosley's research in women's responses to medications was considered eccentric, even irrelevant. "For a long time, I felt lonely," he said in a recent interview. "Other scientists used to say: 'Why are you wasting your time?' It's not a waste of time. Lives have been lost."[4]

In 2001, a U.S. General Accounting Office report ("Drug Safety: Most Drugs Withdrawn in Recent Years Had Greater Health Risks for Women") showed that "eight of the 10 prescription drugs withdrawn since January 1, 1997, posed greater health risks for women than for men."[5] With four of these drugs, the increased risk was clear. With four others, including the diabetes drug Rezulin with which two thirds of the deaths were in women, the increased risk may have been the result of women's greater usage. These findings, according to *The Washington Post*, added weight "to the call for pharmaceutical companies to study whether a drug produces the same side effects in men and women."[6] Although studies begun in the last five years have included more female subjects, few have addressed whether women are responding differently and why. A 1998 study acknowledged this, stating: "For a number of drugs it is well recognized that women suffer more frequently from side-effects, however it is often not clear if this is due to gender differences in the pharmacokinetics [drug metabolism in the body] or pharmacodynamics [how drugs act in the body]. Very little is known about these gender-related differences and the possibility that women may show a different pattern of treatment response than men."[7] By 2001, little had changed. Dr. Woosley told the *Post* that many drug studies he sees "don't consider sex differences at all."[8]

SERIOUS SCRUTINY INTO women's responses to medications is long overdue. A substantially larger percentage of the female population (55 percent) takes a prescription medication daily than the male population (37 percent) in the U.S.[9] Yet, for decades women have ex-perienced tremendous harm from improperly researched and dosed medications. This harm is usually the result of inadequate research and poorly designed drug doses. The birth control pills introduced in America in 1960 contained 300 to 600 percent more estrogen than necessary. Within two years doctors had begun reporting cases of blood clots in the legs (thrombophlebitis), clots moving to the lungs (thromboembolism), strokes, and deaths to the FDA. These and other side effects were dose-related and could have been avoided if the drug companies had taken the time to develop lower, safer doses—just as birth control pills contain today.[10–14]

Instead, it took nearly a decade to clearly establish that the first birth control pills were causing these problems and heart attacks and strokes as well. During this time, millions of women continued to re-ceive high-dose birth control pills, thousands developed severe side effects, and hundreds died.

Even after a decade of this, the FDA had done little to rectify things. Meanwhile, British researchers uncovered the evidence that the high-dose pills were causing hundreds of unnecessary deaths. A study in 1977 by the Royal College of General Practitioners found that "the death-rate from diseases of the circulatory system in women who had used oral contraceptives was five times that of controls who had never used them; and the death-rate in those who had taken the pill continuously for 5 years or more was ten times that of the controls."[15] British doctors also clearly established that low-dose pills were much safer.

In Britain, the authorities didn't hesitate to act. By 1969, doctors were directed to use lower-dose pills, and by 1970 the high-dose pills virtually vanished from the British market. Similar actions in other Eu-ropean countries led to a rapid drop in the number of serious reac-tions involving birth control pills.[16] But in the U.S., rather than act directly to change the methods of the drug companies and doctors, the FDA simply added warnings to the package inserts and notified doctors by letters. Britain considered these interventions and rejected them as too slow and too ineffective. According to historian Lara

Marks, the difference in intervention between Britain and the U.S. was indicative of "the nature of each country's regulatory mechanism and the power pharmaceutical companies could exert over government decisions."[17]

The differences in approach were soon obvious. In 1978, eight years after high-dose pills disappeared from Britain, 40 percent of the ten million American women on birth control pills were being prescribed high doses.[18] In other words, nearly twenty years after the drug industry introduced birth control pills at dangerously high doses, they were still producing and doctors were still prescribing high-dose pills to four million American women.

By the twenty-five-year mark, most American doctors had adapted, but 400,000 American women still received high-dose birth control pills.[19] Most of these women were 35 to 39 years old, when the risks of thrombophlebitis and thromboembolism were highest.

Finally, in 1988, twenty-eight years after the first birth control pills were introduced, high-dose pills were withdrawn from the U.S. market—but the problems weren't over. Birth control pills also contain progestins, another type of powerful hormone. The progestins in the first birth control pills were up to 1,000 percent higher than those used today and were linked to heart attacks, clots in arteries, strokes, and problems with normal blood sugar maintenance. These problems from high-dose progestins were identified later than the problems from high-dose estrogens, and lowering the doses of progestins in birth control pills took even longer. Today, birth control pills contain about one tenth of the amount of progestins than originally, as the FDA itself acknowledges: "Over the years, the amount of estrogen has been reduced by one-third or less of that in the first birth control pills, and the progestin has been decreased to one-tenth or less."[20] This acknowledgment after the fact provides small comfort to the women who took the high-dose pills and, as is now known, have a higher risk of breast cancer.[21,22]

How many thousands of women were harmed by the unnecessarily high doses of estrogens and progestins in birth control pills? No one knows. Why did it take decades after birth control pills were released for widespread usage to figure this out? How could the drug companies and the FDA have approved such unnecessarily high doses in the first place? In 1960 it was known that hormones were extremely potent, side-effect–prone chemicals. Better dose-response studies could have been conducted, and safety could have been better assured. After approval, vigilance should have been provided for these new, potent hormonal drugs. Unfortunately, the monitoring of new drugs was inadequate then, and it remains inadequate today.

SOME DOCTORS BELIEVE the differences in women's and men's responses to medications are mainly due to size, not gender. "Size makes a big difference," a specialist told me. "I adjust doses for smaller patients, who most often are women."

Size certainly is a factor, but not a definitive one. Sometimes a small patient requires big doses, and a large patient tolerates only small ones. Other factors are involved, including age, differing metabolic rates, differences in kidney function, and differences in the person's genetically determined enzyme systems that metabolize drugs in the liver. Genetics also explain a phenomenon I saw in my patients and other doctors have reported in theirs. As one doctor described it: "If their mothers are sensitive to a drug, many of my female patients are sensitive too."

Whatever the reasons, the result is that, in general, women seem to display greater sensitivities and increased responses to medications than men. As a specialist in women's medicine told me two decades ago, "I see a lot of women who are unusually sensitive to medications. While the majority handle standard doses just fine, a surprising number do better and experience fewer side effects with lower doses. When they tell me they're sensitive, I believe them. They know. They've convinced me." Unfortunately, most drugs continue to be recommended at the very same doses for women as for men.

The lack of information about women's responses to medications means that, for now, most of our knowledge will continue to be derived from hindsight—that is, from recognizing medication reactions in women after they occur. This was how Dr. Woosley belatedly discovered women's heightened sensitivity to Seldane. Unfortunately, belated discovery is a wasteful strategy that allows unnecessary harm to occur for years. Because doctors like Woosley are rare and funding is scarce, many medication problems are never discovered or rectified.

Even when such problems are recognized, the current system often fails to respond. Although Seldane's cardiac toxicity was dose-related, a lower, proven-effective dosage was never marketed or recommended. Another example: In 1999 the military was beset by a controversy over its anthrax vaccine. A small percentage of soldiers and physicians claimed that the vaccine was unsafe. Women had the highest rate of reactions to the vaccine. Perhaps this was because the vaccine was not weight-adjusted, so women received the same dosage as men.

The importance of designing drugs for different sizes, ages, and tolerances became apparent again with Redux and Fen-Phen, the weight-loss sensations of the middle 1990's. Many people obtained good results with these drugs, which quickly became hot topics for television programs and magazine articles. Consumers flocked to doctors and clinics offering Redux and Fen-Phen. Billboards appeared advertising Fen-Phen at bargain prices. The drugs became a national obsession.

Then, just as suddenly, Redux's and Fen-Phen's safety came into question. This didn't result from drug company research, but by accident. A medical technician noticed an abnormally high number of rare heart abnormalities in women who were taking Redux or Fen-Phen. She told the doctors, but they dismissed her observations. More women showed up with heart-valve deformities until the trend couldn't be ignored. Further research revealed not only a shocking increase in heart abnormalities—one study found heart valve damage in 33 percent of Redux and Fen-Phen users—but also a marked increase of pulmonary hypertension, a disabling, often lethal condition. Within a year, Redux and Pondimin (one of the two drugs in Fen-Phen) were gone.

Redux and Pondimin had undergone years of intensive research before being approved in the United States. The drugs had been used

in Europe for years. Yet, the serious dangers of these seemingly mirac-
ulous weight-loss drugs weren't discovered until after usage by 6 million Americans, mostly women. Why did these side effects occur?
Perhaps in part because Redux's and Fen-Phen's doses were one-
size-fits-all. All women (and men) got the same dose no matter their
weight, age, or history of reactivity to medications. Women who
weighed 125 pounds got the same dose as women weighing 350
pounds; 65-year-old women got the same dose as 21-year-old men.
Women with other medical conditions and taking several other medications got the same dose as completely healthy women. Such methods court disaster, because they ignore the fundamental medical
principle and everyday clinical fact of individual variation in people's
medication responses.

HOW CAN WOMEN protect themselves from side effects of overmedication? First, by not assuming that a manufacturer-recommended
dose is right for them, and by not letting their doctors assume this, either. Even if a study demonstrates that a majority of women require a
standard dosage of a drug, there still may be many women who don't.
A glaring example is an early study of Motrin published in *Current
Therapeutic Research*.[23] In this study, 25 women preferred 400 mg (every
4 to 6 hours) for controlling menstrual pain and 19 women preferred
only 200 mg. The authors stated "the extent to which the two dosage
levels of ibuprofen afforded relief were not significantly different. In
some women it would seem that 200 mg taken at four-hour intervals
offers significant relief and that a higher dosage may offer little or
no advantage for the treatment of dysmenorrhea." Unfortunately, the
authors didn't stop there: "However, since more women rated the
larger dose [400 mg of Motrin] as most effective, and considering
the relative lack of side effects from the medication, the higher dose
could be chosen for routine prescription." In other words, give every
woman the 400-mg dose, even if 200 mg is all that 42 percent of them
prefer.

Equally questionable is the authors' comment about a "lack of side
effects." Anti-inflammatory drugs like Motrin prompt more side-effect

reports to the FDA than any other group of medications. Gastrointestinal hemorrhaging from anti-inflammatory drugs has led to 70,000 hospitalizations and 16,000 deaths each year for more than a decade.[24] Is it important to use the very lowest effective dose of Motrin? Absolutely. Scores of journal articles and all of the top drug references explicitly recommend using the lowest doses of anti-inflammatory drugs. Even the *PDR* recommends this. Actually, The Upjohn Company recommended the same with Motrin: "The smallest effective dose should be used."

Yet, if a woman goes for treatment of menstrual pain and her physician selects Motrin, he will almost invariably prescribe the 400-mg dose. Very likely he has never seen the data on the effectiveness of low-dose Motrin, because Upjohn has never placed it in the *Physicians' Desk Reference.* Indeed, before the manufacturer decided that developing a 200-mg, over-the-counter dose of Motrin might be profitable, a 200-mg Motrin pill was not available in the United States.

The same pattern is occurring today with Celebrex, the new, top-selling anti-inflammatory drug. Celebrex rises to higher blood levels in older women, producing greater risks of side effects, but Searle doesn't recommend lower doses for this group. Searle does advise doctors: "The lowest dose of Celebrex should be sought for each patient."[25] But the lowest dose Searle recommends for anyone of any age is 100 mg twice daily. For osteoarthritis, Celebrex's most common use, the recommended dose is a one-size-fits-all, 100 mg twice daily for everyone. Searle does not produce or even mention the effectiveness of 50 mg twice daily, a 50 percent lower dosage that was proven effective in a large study conducted by the Mayo Clinic—a study in which more than 70 percent of the subjects were women.[26]

WHEN WOMEN NO longer need contraception, they usually face an even tougher dilemma with the onset of menopause, which often brings hot flashes, burning urination, painful sex, depression, or intense anxiety. Menopause also can bring osteoporosis, with marked increases in the risk of hip and spinal fractures. In the U.S., 1.3 million fractures from osteoporosis occur annually, and women have a two-to-four-times-greater risk than men.[27] By age 85, 33 percent of women have suffered hip fractures,[28] which are a common cause of chronic pain, disability, and ultimately death. According to a 1995 article in the *International Journal of Gynaecology and Obstetrics*, "25% of women who sustain such a fracture will not survive the first year."[29]

But the decision about treating the degenerative changes of menopause may be even more difficult than the decision about contraception had been previously. For four decades the most-used treatment has been hormone replacement therapy. This usually consists of an estrogen medication or a drug containing an estrogen and a progesterone.

The preferred estrogen formulation among doctors is Premarin, which was introduced in 1964. Premarin may be the most prescribed drug ever: It was the most prescribed drug in the U.S. in 1999, when women filled 47,768,000 prescriptions for it.[30] In comparison, Prozac logged 24 million prescriptions. Premarin's popularity is not new: It was also the most prescribed drug every year from 1992 to 1998, and that's as far back as my records go. In addition, Premarin is one of the two hormones in Prempro, the number-fourteen most prescribed drug in 1999 with 21,883,000 prescriptions. In total, 69.5 million prescriptions containing Premarin were filled in 1999.

Premarin is popular in part due to Wyeth-Ayerst's claim that Premarin is "a mixture of estrogens obtained exclusively from natural sources."[31] The "natural" part sounds good to physicians and patients. However, the "natural sources" for Premarin are the estrogens obtained from the urine of mares. These estrogens are indeed natural to horses, but they aren't natural to humans. Side effects with Premarin are common. "I don't know why doctors keep prescribing Premarin and Prempro," a medication expert told me. "In my experience, Premarin causes a lot of side effects, especially depression and mood problems. A lot of women just can't handle Premarin. Premarin and Prempro contain hormones that are not natural to the human body, and this creates problems."

Even a top official at the FDA doesn't seem impressed with Premarin. When asked about Premarin's perennial popularity, Janet Woodcock, director of the FDA's Center for Drug Evaluation and

Research (CDER), replied, "The predominant use of Premarin is a practice pattern of American physicians, probably resulting from advertising."[32]

Estrogens like Premarin can cause many side effects, including fluid retention, breast tenderness, headaches, irritability, vaginal bleeding, blood clots, pulmonary embolism, and strokes. Many women feel worse when taking estrogens like Premarin than when not taking them, and they quit treatment. Up to 50 to 80 percent of women started on hormone therapy for menopause quit within a year.[33–35] Much of this is avoidable, because the side effects with Premarin and other estrogens are dose-related: The higher the dose, the more often and more severe the side effects. Yet for decades, many women have been getting overmedicated with Premarin. From 1964 through 1999, Wyeth-Ayerst recommended an initial dose of 1.25 mg/day of Premarin for treating hot flashes, the menopausal symptom that most often causes women to seek treatment. But by the late 1970's, problems with Premarin side effects led many experts to recommend using half this amount, 0.625 mg/day initially[36–38]—yet, this lower, safer dosage was not reflected in the Premarin package insert or *PDR* dosage guidelines for hot flashes until 2000.

Even this dosage is excessive for treating many women's hot flashes. Studies in *Menopause*[39] and in *Annals of Internal Medicine,*[40] and guidelines in the American Medical Association Drug Evaluations[41] and the *American Hospital Formulary Service, Drug Information,*[42] indicate that as little as 0.3 mg of Premarin is often effective and better tolerated with some women.

Wyeth-Ayerst's recommended dosages for preventing osteoporosis have also been high. From 1974 through 1987, the company recommended 1.25 mg of Premarin for preventing osteoporosis. Yet, studies throughout the 1970's and early 1980's showed that half this amount was sufficient.[43–46] By the time Wyeth-Ayerst reduced the recommended dosage to 0.625 mg in 1988, a study in the *Annals of Internal Medicine* in 1987 had already shown that just 0.3 mg of Premarin, with calcium and vitamin D or combined with progesterone, was sufficient.[47] Subsequent studies in the *American Journal of Medicine,*[48]

Annals of Internal Medicine,[49] *JAMA,*[50] *Maturitas,*[51] and *Menopause*[52] confirmed the effectiveness of 0.3 mg/day of Premarin with calcium and vitamin D or soy protein.

In fact, in one study involving 130 women ages 55 and over who were taking standard doses of estrogen, 95 percent were able to switch to a one-half dosage while still obtaining satisfactory control of menopausal symptoms.[53] These findings indicate not only that low-dose estrogen works, but that many women today taking standard Premarin doses may be getting overmedicated.

Daily doses of 0.3 mg, 0.625 mg, and 1.25 mg of Premarin all sound small. In fact, the 108-percent increase from 0.3 to 0.625 is very large pharmacologically, and the 408-percent increase from 0.3 to 1.25 mg is enormous. Remember, estrogens are some of the most potent chemicals on the planet. Doubling or quadrupling a dosage can increase the risks, which is important to know because the estrogens and particularly the progesterones in the hormonal treatment of menopausal symptoms have now been linked with higher rates of breast cancer, and estrogens have also now been linked with increases in ovarian cancer.[54-59]

Other popular types of estrogens such as Estratab (esterified estrogens), Estrace (oral estradiol), and Estraderm (transdermal estradiol) have also been proven effective for treating hot flashes at doses at least 50 percent lower than recommended by their manufacturers.[60-70] (See Table 5.1, page 85). Furthermore, the progesterone (medroxyprogesterone) contained in combination pills such as Prempro is synthetic and associated with many side effects. Progesterones do improve bone strength and block estrogen's cancer-causing effects on the uterus, but they can also cause irritability, emotional instability, headaches, fluid retention, bloating, weight gain, facial hair, and acne. These side effects are dose-related. Premarin itself is made in a lower-dose pill (0.3 mg), but the lowest amount of Premarin in Prempro remains 0.625 mg.

With today's hormone replacement therapy causing so many dose-related side effects, is it any wonder that so many women quit treatment? But quitting or avoiding treatment is not a good solution for women having severe hot flashes, or unable to have sex because of vaginal pain, or risking fractures from osteoporosis. The average woman spends a third of her life over age fifty. For most women, menopause is a hormone deficiency disorder that has serious consequences. When the treatment is properly fitted to the individual, women report feeling much better, and they enjoy better, healthier lives.

This is why overmedicating women with unnecessarily high doses of Premarin and Prempro and other hormones for menopause is so regrettable, for it not only makes them feel miserable but drives millions of women from vital treatment and causes many others to be fearful of getting treatment.[71, 72] This is why Dr. Bruce Ettinger, a leading researcher in hormonal therapy, stated in 1993: "I suspect that many more women would choose to continue with long-term estrogen treatment if they used a low-dosage regimen."[73] In 1999 he added: "It is now time to replace the widely held belief that less than the standard dosage of estrogen is without benefit. . . . Long-term continuance of hormonal treatment therapy may be improved if lower dosages are given, particularly if the regimen is tailored to the needs of the patient."[74]

Alternate drugs for preventing osteoporosis such as Evista (raloxifene) and Fosamax (alendronate) offer advantages—and different risks. Evista appears not only to prevent osteoporosis, but also to reduce markedly the risk of breast cancer.[75] Evista, however, mimics some of the effects of estrogens and can cause thrombophlebitis and strokes. Also, Evista can provoke or worsen hot flashes, which already occur in 50 to 80 percent of premenopausal women.

Fosamax is very effective for preventing osteoporosis, but it can be terribly irritating to the esophagus and stomach. Severe heartburn is common. The medical literature contains more than a dozen reports of severe scorching of the esophagus, some of which required surgical correction. A 2000 study has shown that Fosamax is almost as irritating to the stomach as anti-inflammatory drugs. When Fosamax and anti-inflammatory drugs were used together, 30 percent of study subjects got gastric ulcers.[76] Actonel, a new drug related to Fosamax, may also cause heartburn, esophagitis, or gastric ulcers.

With both Fosamax and Evista, which many women will take for decades, the long-term risks are unknown. Thus, it is important to use the lowest, safest dosage. However, Evista is one-size-fits-all. For preventing osteoporosis, so is Fosamax.

BECAUSE THE RACE to develop and market new drugs is so profit-driven, other useful alternatives are often neglected. For example, estrogens and progesterones can be derived from vegetables and fashioned into hormones that are identical to those natural to women. Multiple reports suggest that these natural hormones cause fewer side effects and are tolerated better than Premarin and Prempro:

- *Infertility and Reproductive Medicine Clinics of North America,* 1995: "Better compliance, because of little breakthrough bleeding, with the natural regimen."[77]
- *International Journal of Fertility and Women's Medicine,* 1997: "Synthetic estrogens and progestins, as found in oral contraceptives, tend to elevate blood pressure, while naturally occurring estrogens lower it, or have no effect."[78]
- *Obstetrics and Gynecology,* 1989: "We and others have demonstrated that a micronized natural progesterone preparation administered orally can produce excellent blood levels without the unwanted effects (such as fluid retention, breast tenderness, weight gain, and depression) of the synthetics."[79]
- *Fertility and Sterility,* 1999: "In addition to the decreased potential for adverse effects [with natural hormones], there are clear advantages in convenience, cost, compliance, and quality of life."[80]

I know several women who had miserable times with drug company hormones, yet have done very well with natural hormones. The most common adverse effect is sedation; as always, tailoring the dose to the individual is the key. Natural estrogens come in several forms. Best known among mainstream doctors are Estrace and other forms of estradiol, which are oral medications, and Estraderm, a skin patch. Women may require doses from 0.25 to 2 mg orally or from 0.05 to 0.1 mg of the skin patch. As a 1995 study advised, "The estradiol dose should be titrated on an individual basis."[81]

Estriol, the mildest estrogen, is commonly used in Europe, but most American physicians don't know about it because it can't be patented and therefore doesn't receive drug company backing and advertising, which have great influence on which drugs doctors prescribe. Estriol is the predominant type of estrogen used by compounding pharmacies in fashioning combinations matched to women's natural estrogen balance. One preparation, Tri-Est, contains a ratio of 80 percent estriol, 10 percent estradiol, 10 percent estrone. Another contains 80 percent estriol and 20 percent estradiol. The most common dosages are 1.25 or 2.5 mg twice daily, but some women need only 0.625 mg twice daily while others need 5 mg twice daily. Even with natural hormones, individual variation plays a major role.

THE FINAL CHAPTER on treating menopausal symptoms such as hot flashes and vaginal atrophy and on preventing osteoporosis has not been written. New approaches and new drugs seem to arrive yearly—and each poses the challenge to translate information and dosages based on broad studies and statistics into treatment designed to match individual women's needs.

Nor has the final chapter been written on the effects of other medications in women. Indeed, with several major groups of drugs, we are just beginning to consider the possibility that women's responses may differ from men's. For example, every five years a blue-ribbon panel of experts on hypertension—the Joint National Committee on the Detection, Evaluation, and Treatment of High Blood Pressure (JNC)—convenes, reviews recent advances, and issues a comprehensive summary of issues and interventions for treating hypertension. Among the interventions, the committee lists the preferred antihypertensive drugs and their dosages. In March 2001, I published an article in the *Archives of Internal Medicine* comparing the antihypertensive drug doses recommended by the JNC and the doses recommended by the drug companies.[82] For 23 of 40 medications (58 percent), the drug companies' recommended initial doses were substantially higher than those recommended by the JNC. For 22 drugs, the drug company initial doses were at least 100 percent higher.

Perhaps not coincidentally, researchers have reported higher incidences of some adverse effects in women taking antihypertensive drugs.[83,84] Thus, one author commented in the *American Journal of the Medical Sciences:* "Antihypertensive-associated side effects that seem to occur more frequently in women than in men could be due to the fact that women are treated with antihypertensives using the dosage and schedule established with men, even though it is well known that body size, fat distribution, and coronary artery size differ in women and men."[85]

WHEN THE FDA removed over-the-counter diet remedies containing phenylpropanolamine, it was mainly because of risks to women. *The New York Times* reported: "The Yale study found an increased risk of a certain type of stroke, hemorrhagic stroke, among women who had taken appetite suppressants containing phenylpropanolamine, and among women who were first-time users of the drug."[86]

IN SOME STUDIES of cholesterol-lowering drugs, women have also shown greater responses and more side effects when given the same dosages as men.[87–90] In one study involving Baycol, women obtained a significantly greater reduction in low-density lipoprotein cholesterol (LDL–C) with 0.4 mg of the drug than men, 44.4 percent to 37.0 percent.[91] When women were given one half the dosage, their LDL–C reduction of 35.4 percent almost equaled the reduction achieved by men at the full dosage. With the lower dosage, side effects were fewer, and fewer patients quit treatment. Other studies have not found differences in responses to cholesterol-lowering drugs between men and women, so further study is warranted. However, lower doses of cholesterol-lowering drugs have been effective in reaching preferred cholesterol levels for both women and men with mild to moderate cholesterol elevations and without heart disease. Obtaining proper treatment for elevated cholesterol is important because, as stated in a 2001 article in the *Archives of Internal Medicine*, "Cardiovascular disease, primarily coronary heart disease, outnumbers the next 16 causes of death [including all cancers) in women combined. . . . Women are 4 to 8 times more likely to die of cardiovascular disease than of any other disease. . . ."[92] Over the decades, coronary disease has been considered less serious and therefore has been less vigorously treated in women. This is misguided. Women beyond menopause should be evaluated and treated for cholesterol disorders as aggressively as men. However, this doesn't mean overly aggressive drug therapy—it simply means proper therapy, as explained in the next chapter.

Clearly, more research is needed into the differences in drug response between women and men, but progress has been slow. An April 2000 headline from *The New York Times* News Service read: "Sex Bias Found in Medical Research." The article began: "Health care for women may suffer because researchers overlook important differences between the sexes in clinical trials evaluating new methods of treating or preventing disease, experts say."[93] One year later, an article in *The New York Times* was reporting the same thing: "The National Academy of Sciences said today that biomedical research should pay more attention to differences between men and women in diseases and treatments. Sex differences are pervasive, the academy's report stated."[94] The National Academy of Sciences panel wrote, "The cells of males and females have many basic biochemical differences, and many of these stem from genetic rather than hormonal differences." The panel added that in the past, medical researchers often viewed men as the norm while tending to "underreport rather than highlight sex differences." This tendency, the panel said, "can still be found in the current medical literature."[95]

AS THIS CHAPTER has shown, one important difference between women and men that remains to be recognized and understood is in dose response. With which drugs do differences in dose response occur? How might physicians and patients better anticipate these differences? It will be years before these questions are answered and

84

medication doses are designed properly. Even then, no guarantee exists that the methods used will be any better than the industry's shotgun methods today. Now and in the future, using the lowest, safest doses of medications is almost always the best approach for nonacute conditions and especially for the long-term treatment of women as well as men.

TABLE 5.1

Eight of the Ten Drugs Withdrawn by the FDA Since January 1997 Posed Greater Risks for Women

Drug	Usage	Date Approved	Date Withdrawn	Risk
Pondimin* (fenfluramine)	appetite suppressant	6/14/73	9/15/97	heart valve disease
Redux* (dexfenfluramine)	appetite suppressant	4/29/96	9/15/97	heart valve disease
Seldane (terfenadine)	antihistamine	5/8/85	2/27/98	cardiac arrhythmias
Posicor (mibefradil)	cardiovascular drug	6/20/97	6/8/98	low heart rate in elderly, multiple drug interactions
Hismanal (astemizole)	antihistamine	12/19/88	6/18/99	cardiac arrhythmias
Rezulin* (troglitazone)	diabetes	1/29/97	3/21/00	liver failure
Propulsid (cisapride)	gastrointestinal	7/29/93	7/14/00	cardiac arrhythmias
Lotronex* (alosetron)	gastrointestinal	2/9/00	11/28/00	impaired intestinal blood flow

*Increased risk in women may be a reflection of greater usage with women patients.

Adapted from: Heinrich, J, Director. Health Care—Public Health Issues, United States General Accounting Office. "Drug Safety: Most Drugs Withdrawn in Recent Years Had Greater Health Risks for Women." Letter to Senators Harkin, Snowe, Mikulski. GAO-01-286R Drugs Withdrawn from Market, Jan. 19, 2001.

TABLE 5.2

Effective Low-Dose Hormones for Treating Hot Flashes

These lower doses are effective for many women, but like all medications, the dose must be tailored to be individual. Starting low reduces the number and severity of side effects.

	Drug Company's Recommended Dose (mg)	Effective Lower Dose (mg)
ESTROGENS		
Premarin (conjugated estrogens)		
1964–1999	1.25 (1964–1999)	0.3–0.625[96–98]
Today	0.625 (2000)	0.3[99–102]
Estratab (esterified estrogens)	1.25	0.3–0.625[103–104]
Estrace (oral estradiol) (Estradiol is also available as a generic.)	1–2	0.5[105–107]
Estraderm (Transdermal estradiol is about 20 times more potent than oral estradiol. A 0.05-mg daily dose of transdermal estradiol = 1 mg/day of oral estradiol.)	0.05–0.1	0.02–0.025[108–110]
COMBINATIONS		
Prempro conjugated estrogens with medroxyprogesterone	0.625 2.5	0.3 2.5

Adapted from: Cohen, J.S. "Do Standard Doses of Frequently Prescribed Drugs Cause Preventable Adverse Effects in Women?" Accepted for publication by the *Journal of the American Medical Women's Association*, April 2001.

This listing is for information purposes only. Readers should not change drugs or dosages unless specifically directed to do so by their own doctors.

TABLE 5.3

Is the Hormone You Are Taking Really Natural?

Although many types of hormones are called "natural," only those composed entirely of estradiol, estrone, or estriol—the three types of estrogens naturally produced by women—are truly natural for women.

	Type of Estrogen	Identical to Human Estrogens
ESTROGENS		
Drug-Company Products		
Premarin conjugated estrogens (0.3, 0.625, 0.9, 1.25, 2.5 mg)	equilin, 17-dihydrequilin, and estrone	no no yes
Estratab (0.3, 0.625, 1.25, 2.5 mg)	equilin and estrone	no yes
Ogen, Ortho-Est (0.75, 1.5, 3, 6 mg)	estropipate	no
Estinyl (0.02, 0.05 mg)	ethinyl estradiol	no
Estrace (0.05, 1, 2 mg)	estradiol (oral)	yes
Estraderm, Climara 0.05 and 0.1 mg/day	estradiol (transdermal)	yes
*Compounding Pharmacy Products**		
Natural Estriol estriol: 1, 2 mg twice daily	estriol	yes
Triple Natural Estrogen 80% estriol, 10% estradiol, 10% estrone (0.625, 1.25, 2.5, 5 mg twice daily)	all 3 estrogens	yes
Dual Natural Estrogen 80% estriol, 20% estradiol (0.625, 1.25, 2.5, 5 mg twice daily)	estriol/estradiol	yes
PROGESTERONES		
Drug-Company Products		
Medroxyprogesterone Provera, others: 2.5, 5, 10 mg		no
*Compounding Pharmacy Products**		
Natural Micronized Progesterone progesterone: 50, 100, 200 mg twice daily		yes

COMBINATION PILLS**

Drug-Company Products

Conjugated Estrogens and Medroxyprogesterone Prempro, Premphase: Premarin 0.625 mg and Provera 2.5, 5 mg	no

Compounding Pharmacy Products*

Mixtures of the above natural estrogens and progesterones are individualized.

* These non-patented products are made by compounding pharmacies, which upon receiving physicians' orders will mail the prescriptions to patients. These products are not generally available in regular pharmacies.

** Although a combination pill is slightly more convenient, a better choice of hormones and more precise dosing can be accomplished with separate estrogen and progesterone products.

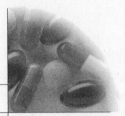

Why 50 to 75 Percent of People Quit Taking Their Cholesterol-Lowering Medications

ARE NEEDLESS SIDE effects limited to a few drugs—Prozac, Voltaren, Motrin, Celebrex, Viagra, birth control pills, Redux, Fen-Phen, Premarin, Provera—or is this a systemic problem involving scores of drugs and millions of people? This chapter will answer this question by discussing one of the most important, most frequently prescribed groups of medications today: cholesterol-lowering drugs.

During the 1990s, there were few areas of medication therapy where confusion reigned as much as with cholesterol-lowering drugs. Controversy and confusion abounded about who should be treated for high cholesterol, how vigorously they should be treated, and which drugs and dosages should be used. A new report by the National Cholesterol Education Program (NCEP) on detecting and treating cholesterol problems should clarify some of these issues.[1] However, questions still remain about whether many people with mild-to-moderate cholesterol elevations need medication treatment, and as usual, about the intensity of medication treatment, especially initially.

Getting proper treatment for high cholesterol is crucial. Coronary heart disease remains our number-one killer and strokes are number three, and the leading cause of both is the atherosclerosis associated with high cholesterol. What can slow, stop, and even reverse atherosclerosis? Reducing cholesterol, especially the type of cholesterol known as low-density–lipoprotein cholesterol, or LDL-C, the preferred measurement for assessing risk. What medications best reduce LDL-C? The six cholesterol-lowering drugs known as the "statins"— Lipitor, Zocor, Pravachol, Mevacor, Baycol, Lescol. The statins constitute one of the most successful medication groups of all time. In 1999, nearly 100,000,000 prescriptions were filled for these six drugs, generating nearly $8 billion in sales.

Yet, statin and other lipid-lowering drugs have failed as many patients as they've helped. "Approximately 50% of patients placed on a lipid-lowering drug quit taking the drug in one year, and only 25% still take the drug two years after it was started," Dr. William Roberts, the editor in chief of the *American Journal of Cardiology,* reported in his highly respected journal. "Thus, we have available five [now six] drugs that have the capacity to prevent and arrest atherosclerosis, but few patients who need them are on them."[2]

Why do people motivated enough to seek treatment and to start taking medications decide to discontinue? One major reason is side effects. "Most people I see on statins get side effects," one pharmacist, preferring anonymity, told me. "The side effects usually are muscle discomfort or gastrointestinal problems, and they don't seem to diminish with time. Sooner or later, people get tired of the side effects and stop taking their medication."

Many of these side effects are dose-related and could be avoided by matching statin dosages to patients' tolerances. But the trend among many doctors today is to use the most powerful statins at doses that are higher than many patients need, as Shirley's case illustrates:

In May 1998, my doctor suggested I take Lipitor. After I checked it out, it seemed safe. However, I had a bad reaction to it, and by the time my doctor was convinced Lipitor was the problem (it was the only thing I was taking), I was so ill, it took over a year for me to recover.

Shirley's side effects included pain in several joints, swelling of the legs, twinges in fingers and arms, painful muscles, and weakness. The doctor assured her the Lipitor wasn't the cause. When the symptoms didn't abate, he prescribed an anti-inflammatory drug for the pain. Finally, he discontinued the medications. Her improvement was slow. Even after she recovered, the experience still had its consequences.

"I am 66 and have been blessed with good health all of my life until this episode. Now I wonder if I am okay if I get a sniffle. I refuse to take anything now: I have my health back and won't jeopardize it again."

Did Shirley need treatment? Shirley's blood cholesterol level was 230 milligrams/deciliter (mg/dl), which is moderately above the recommended range. Still, because she was 66 years old and healthy, some doctors might have foregone treatment, but others like Shirley's physician would have recommended it.

How much treatment did Shirley require? For people without prior histories of cardiovascular disorders, current guidelines recommend a total cholesterol below 200 mg/dl. To reach this goal, Shirley required a 14-percent reduction in her total blood cholesterol. Yet, some physicians recommend more stringent guidelines, including a total cholesterol of less than 180 mg/dl, which for Shirley would have necessitated a 22-percent reduction.

Shirley's physician chose Lipitor, the most potent statin and the most prescribed cholesterol-lowering drug in the U.S. In 2000, doctors wrote 48,791,000 prescriptions for Lipitor, generating more than $4 billion for Pfizer.[3] But the recommended initial dose of Lipitor is a one-size-fits-all 10 mg for everyone, and by reducing total cholesterol by 29 percent on average, it was excessive for Shirley's needs. This was proven when Shirley's cholesterol level dropped from 230 to 145 mg/dl, which was too much too quickly, and the result was intolerable side effects and another patient quitting treatment.

A one-half dosage of Lipitor (5 mg), which reduces total cholesterol by 21 to 22 percent on average,[4,5] would have been enough for Shirley. Indeed, Lipitor is so powerful that one-half and one-quarter doses (5 and 2.5 mg) are as effective as the standard starting doses of three other top-selling statins: Lescol, Mevacor, and Pravachol.[6]

Why did Shirley's doctor prescribe Lipitor at the full, 10-mg dosage? Because that's what Pfizer recommends for everyone. The Lipitor dosage guidelines do not distinguish between patients with or without heart disease. They do not distinguish between patients requiring large reductions and those needing small reductions. The recommended initial dose of Lipitor, 10 mg, is so powerful that doctors can treat many patients with the same dose and not have to bother matching the dose to individual patients. Ease-of-usage sells.

WHY NOT PRODUCE and recommend lower doses of Lipitor? When Lipitor was introduced in 1997, the market was already cornered by highly successful, more proven rivals like Zocor, Pravachol, and Mevacor. Marketing Lipitor successfully was a challenge. "The drugs are all relatively similar," Dr. David Waters, chief of cardiology at San Francisco General Hospital, told *The New York Times*. "Whether one sells better than another really depends on marketing, first of all. . . ."[7] Pfizer met this challenge by producing Lipitor at an initial dose so potent in reducing cholesterol that many patients wouldn't need any dose increases, thus allowing Pfizer to market Lipitor as easy-to-use for physicians. "72% of patients reached their National Cholesterol Education Program LDL-C goal at 10 mg," Lipitor advertising boasts.[8] Lipitor's sales zoomed past all of the better-known statins. Now television advertising for Lipitor boasts its power in reducing cholesterol, and sales have jumped even further.

However, more is not necessarily better with medications. A pot of coffee probably satisfies the needs of 72 percent of coffee drinkers, but that doesn't mean they all should drink that much. With Lipitor and other statin drugs, as with all types of cholesterol-lowering drugs, most side effects are dose-related.[9,10] Higher doses increase the risks and contribute to the 38 to 75 percent of people who quit cholesterol-lowering medications.[11–14]

"I know doctors who go around claiming that these drugs are harmless, that no dosage is too high," a researcher at the University of California, San Diego, told me. "They just refuse to see the dangers or recognize the problems—or that we have no idea how these drugs will affect people after ten or twenty years. The whole situation is out of control." This doctor is so concerned, that he has begun investigating several types of statin side effects. "We get so many patients who have obvious side effects to statin drugs yet are told by their doctors that it isn't the medication. These are people who have never had these types of problems before. These people go from doctor to doctor, seeking help. When they finally get to us, they are so relieved, they say, 'Thank God someone understands that it isn't in my head.'"

The doctor has received many cases as severe as Shirley's. "For some people, the side effects take weeks or months to go away. For some, they still haven't gone away."

"There is no question that these drugs are miracle drugs. They save millions of lives every year," Dr. Paul Phillips, a cardiologist at Scripps Mercy Hospital in San Diego, told the *San Diego Union-Tribune*. "What irks me is, it's important to know all sides of the equation, and nobody's paying attention to the toxic side of the equation."[15]

Others aren't convinced. "The anxiety about side effects is exaggerated, to say the least," said Dr. Daniel Steinberg, an endocrinologist and co-director of UCSD's Lipid Research Clinic. "These drugs are safer than aspirin. There have been scads of studies that are carefully controlled, and any effects are noted."[16]

However, Dr. Beatrice Golomb, of UCSD, told the newspaper, "I deeply believe that it's important that somebody take an honest look at it . . . that isn't being funded by the pharmaceutical industry." For this purpose, she has received a $4 million grant from the National Institutes of Health.[17]

Less debatable is the fact that by May 2000 the FDA received ninety cases of liver failure and more than thirty deaths related to statin drugs.[18] Thirteen liver failure cases and nine deaths were linked with Lipitor. In response, the FDA has recommended the addition of warnings to statin package inserts about the possibility of liver failure.[19]

Liver injury from statins is dose-related. At low doses, statins cause no more liver abnormalities than placebos. But according to the American Journal of Cardiology: "With each doubling of the dose, the frequency of [significant] liver enzyme elevations . . . also doubles."[20]

Deaths from other causes besides liver injury have been reported, too. In May 2000, this testimony was presented at an FDA public hearing:

> On Oct. 7, 1999, at the age of 48, Elinosa C., a registered nurse, wife and mother, succumbed to the end stages of irreversible dermatomyositis and interstitial pulmonary fibrosis directly caused by her use of a prescribed cholesterol-lowering medication, simvastatin (Zocor). [The cause was confirmed by her physician and a medical examiner, stated the family's attorney, who is also a Harvard-trained physician.] Mrs. Calabio had no substantial risk factors for heart disease. Her cholesterol was slightly high, but not considered dangerous. . . . Clearly, cholesterol lowering drugs are no less potent than any of the many prescribed medications that can kill if improperly used or even when used according to the manufacturers' directions.[21]

This woman's cholesterol was only modestly elevated, requiring 10 mg of Zocor based on study results, but her physician started her on 40 mg. Indeed, she may not have needed treatment at all. The National Cholesterol Education Program states that for premenopausal women with mild cholesterol elevations, "drug therapy should be delayed."[22] Many experts do not treat mild to moderate cholesterol elevations in women until they are at least 55 years old.

USING STATINS SAFELY is important for another reason: Experience with statins is limited, long-term safety is not proven, and yet, many people will take statin medications for life. In a 2000 issue of the British Medical Journal, the authors acknowledged that "seven years is not long enough to eliminate concerns about long-term adverse effects such as cancer."[23] With newer statins such as Lipitor and Baycol, our experience is even more limited. In a September 2000 interview in *The New York Times,* cardiologist Michael Criqui commented that although we have had some good experience with statins, at least twenty years is necessary for assuring long-term safety. Dr. Matthew Muldoon, a cholesterol researcher at the University of Pittsburgh, added, "We have studies that show statins don't cause cancer within a five-year period. Of course, neither does smoking."[24]

Citing the lack of long-term safety data, the National Cholesterol Education Program states that patients "must be well informed about the goals and side effects of the medication."[25] However, Pfizer doesn't provide any information in its package insert or the *PDR* about the effectiveness and reduced risks of low-dose Lipitor, and it doesn't produce low-dose pills. Physicians have to discover the effectiveness of low-dose Lipitor on their own.

Charles was 67 when his doctor prescribed Lipitor at the standard 10-mg dose. When Charles's muscles began to ache, his doctor told him to split the pill in half. The aching stopped, and three months later, Charles's LDL-C had dropped from 187 to 103—a 45-percent reduction with just 5 mg of Lipitor.

Charles's response to low-dose Lipitor is not surprising. Although drug companies only provide information about "average" cholesterol reductions, the variability in response between patients is quite large. A 2000 study in the *American Journal of Cardiology* found: "Individual variation in LDL-C response to statin therapy is large (range 10% to 70%)."[26]

Many patients can obtain excellent responses with low-dose statins—if their physicians remember that individual variation should be considered whenever prescribing any medication.

But physicians who believe in the aggressive use of statins don't agree. Dr. Roberts suggests: "The 'starting dose' . . . should be the one necessary to achieve the goal, not the lowest available dose."[27] Basing the starting dose on statistical averages works for many patients, but it does not ensure that people receive the lowest possible doses to achieve their target cholesterol levels. Individual variation in response to statin drugs is wide, and many people obtain larger reductions than the averages that are reported in package inserts and the *PDR*. For people who are interested in using the lowest, least side-effect prone statin doses, the only way to identify their proper dosage is to start low and, if necessary, increase gradually.

However, using statistical averages to gauge the initial doses of statin drugs will lead to some patients receiving initial doses even higher than recommended in the *PDR*. On the other hand, based on Dr. Roberts's guidelines, physicians should be scaling back from the manufacturer-recommended initial doses for many people with mild to moderate cholesterol elevations—but usually they don't. Instead, they prescribe the standard dosages recommended by statin manu-facturers. The results are cases like Shirley's and Charles's.

Certainly, Dr. Roberts's concerns about patients who do not cur-rently receive adequate treatment with statin drugs is legitimate. In-adequate treatment is just as undesirable as overtreatment. The reality is that with statins, as with all medications, some patients need standard doses, some need higher doses, and some only need lower doses. Drug company guidelines and physicians' methods should ad-dress these differences, thereby reassuring reluctant patients that they will receive the correct amount of medication that each of them needs.

There is another benefit of using low-dose statins: When his doctor reduced his dosage to one half of a pill, Charles's costs for the Lipitor, a very expensive drug, were also halved.

OTHERS HAVE QUESTIONED the trend toward aggressive treat-ment with statin drugs. In a 1997 study titled "Cholesterol reduction and clinical benefit: Are there limits to our expectations?" the re-searchers reported: "About two-thirds of the predictable coronary heart disease incidence can be reversed by a 20% to 35% reduction in LDL cholesterol." Indeed, the greatest reduction in coronary events occurred with the first 5 to10 percent of LDL-C reduction; higher re-ductions produced diminishing degrees of improvement. The au-thors concluded: "The mean reduction [of LDL-C] does not have to be extreme" for patients with mild to moderate hypercholesterolemia and no histories of coronary disease.[28]

The Cholesterol and Recurrent Events (CARE) study involving these types of patients revealed that the rate of coronary events declined as medication treatment reduced LDL-C from 174 to 125 mg/dl, "but no further decline was seen in the LDL range from 125 to 71."[29] In other words, reducing LDL-C to 125 mg/dl is satisfactory for this population. Reaching this level is often possible with low-dose statins.

The authors of the extensive West of Scotland Coronary Prevention Study (WOSCOPS) confessed surprise that the aggressive lowering of LDL-C had limited benefits for patients without coronary disease. "We hypothesized that larger decreases in LDL-C would be associated with greater benefit. However, no clear, graded relationship was observed." A reduction in LDL-C of only 24 percent provided "the full benefit of a 45% risk reduction" of coronary heart disease. They added, "further decreases in LDL were not associated with larger reduction in coronary heart disease risk. . . . a fall in the range of 24% [in LDL-C] is sufficient to produce the full benefit in patients."[30]

These surprising results were mirrored in the studies conducted with low doses of Pravachol and Mevacor when their manufacturers sought FDA approval for over-the-counter preparations of these drugs. Although the applications were denied because of safety concerns, the effectiveness of these low doses in people without cardiovascular disease was impressive. In the study of Pravachol in people with LDL-Cs of 130-190 mg/dl, a low dose of 10 mg allowed 83 percent of subjects to reach the National Cholesterol Education Program's goal of an LDL-C below 160 mg/dl.[31]

The four studies of low-dose Mevacor were even more impressive. These studies involved men over 45 years old and women over 55 with total cholesterol levels between 200 and 240 and LDL-Cs between 130 and 160 mg/dl. Diet counseling and just 10 mg of Mevacor reduced total cholesterol below 200 mg/dl in 45 to 55 percent of these people, and it reduced LDL-C below 130 in 69 to 75 percent. Indeed, 17 to 26 percent achieved an LDL-C below 100 mg/dl.[32]

When these studies are considered with the hundreds of others involving statin drugs, a less than crystal clear picture emerges. For now, for people with cardiovascular disease or diabetes, the target LDL-C of 100 mg/dl recommended by the National Cholesterol Education Program should be heeded. For people without cardiovascular disease but with multiple risk factors and a higher overall risk of having a heart attack, the NCEP guidelines should be seriously considered. However, the CARE and WOSCOP studies suggest that for patients who cannot tolerate statin doses that would accomplish this goal, lesser reductions are indeed worthwhile. Aggressive therapy, even when appropriate, doesn't mean that statin treatment must always be started at aggressive doses. Many people obtain LDL-C reductions that are greater than the average. Dose titration is the key to arriving at the proper dosage for each person and for avoiding side effects that might interfere with treatment.

For the vast majority of people with elevated cholesterol—people without cardiovascular disease or diabetes and with mild-to-moderate cholesterol elevations and few risk factors—statin treatment may not be necessary at all if people eat healthy diets and exercise regularly. Indeed, several experts, including Dr. Walter Willett, professor of epidemiology and nutrition at the Harvard School of Public Health, and Dr. Robert Atkins, the diet guru, expressed concerns that while the new NCEP guidelines suggested nearly tripling the number of people taking statins from 13 million to 36 million, inadequate emphasis was placed on diet and exercise.[33] Certainly, if statin therapy is required for people with mild-to-moderate cholesterol disorders, low-dose statins may provide all of the treatment that is needed.

DESPITE THE FINDINGS of the low-dose studies, the doses that drug companies advise doctors to prescribe continue to creep higher. Zocor was the second most prescribed statin and the fifth best-selling drug overall in America in 1999, when physicians wrote 19,897,000 prescriptions for Zocor, earning $2,305,000,000 for Merck. Merck originally recommended Zocor at an initial dose of 10 mg, but in 1998 it doubled the recommended dose to 20 mg daily. This increase may have been warranted for people with coronary disease or severely elevated levels of cholesterol, but the 10-mg dosage, which reduces LDL-C by 30 percent,[34] is ample for milder cases. Indeed, just 5 mg/day of Zocor reduces LDL-C by 24 percent—enough for more than one third of all people with elevated cholesterol. Independent studies confirm the effectiveness of 5 and 10 mg/day of Zocor, and even as little as 2.5 mg/day in a small percentage of people.[35-37] In one of these studies, 45 percent of patients taking just 5 mg/day of Zocor achieved LDL-C levels of 130 or less, and 59 percent of those taking 10 mg/day of Zocor achieved these levels.[38]

Still, Merck's dosage guidelines recommend 20 mg of Zocor as the preferred starting dose without differentiating between people who have cardiovascular disease and people who don't.[39] This is an important distinction in gauging treatment, but it isn't mentioned in the dosage guidelines of many cholesterol-lowering drugs. At least, farther down in the Zocor dosage guidelines, Merck does state that a lower dose of 10 mg may be enough for moderate LDL-C reductions, and that the recommended dosage range is 5 to 80 mg/day. Merck also provides a chart that shows the effectiveness of 5-mg, 10-mg, and higher doses of Zocor. But do doctors notice? Not the doctor who prescribed Zocor to a 43-year-old man with elevated cholesterol. The man had no cardiovascular disease and only one risk factor, and his LDL-C level required a reduction of 30 percent. A 10-mg-a-day dosage of Zocor reduces LDL-C 30 percent, but instead his physician prescribed 40 mg of Zocor. The man obtained another opinion and responded satisfactorily to a lower Zocor dosage.

Such methods may explain almost weekly letters about side effects with Lipitor and Zocor to the *Los Angeles Times* "People's Pharmacy" column by Joe and Theresa Graedon. These are typical:

"My husband was supposed to take Zocor for a month and then have a cholesterol test. Before the month was up, he developed muscle pains and became very weak. We thought he was getting the flu, but when he was almost paralyzed, we called the emergency room. He was in the hospital for 10 days with a reaction to Zocor that damaged his liver, muscles, kidneys, and eyesight."[40]

"Last fall my doctor prescribed Lipitor, and after several months I found I was having trouble remembering names and coming up with the right word. At dinner once, I said, 'Please pass the elephant,' though I wanted the bread. I told my husband that I thought I'd had a stroke. In January, a friend came to visit. She was worried about her memory and couldn't think of her daughter's name on the telephone. She too was on Lipitor. I asked my doctor to prescribe a different cholesterol medicine. Within a couple of weeks I was more mentally alert. But my friend (still on Lipitor) was in worse shape and afraid she would lose her job. Her doctor said forgetfulness could not be due to the drug. She finally stopped taking Lipitor and now is much sharper."[41]

"I've heard that cholesterol-lowering drugs cause muscle pain and other side effects. I've taken Lopid, Mevacor, Pravachol, and Zocor. I am suffering! My muscles feel so weak I find it hard to walk. It is really difficult to step into the car or even get into the bathtub. Each time I complain about side effects, the doctor writes me a new prescription. I am fed up with these drugs."[42]

These reactions are dose-related. Proper initial doses—indeed, just the simple recognition of obvious statin side effects—would have prevented or minimized these people's reactions.

How might you know if you are responsive to low-dose Lipitor, Zocor, or other statin drugs? Easy: by starting low and, if necessary, increasing gradually. In other words, by working with a doctor who recognizes the importance of matching the dosage to the individual. Not only does this reduce the risk of side effects for people sensitive to these drugs, but it also reduces problems for people who ultimately require high dosages, because their bodies are given adequate time to adjust to the drug, and because they are assured that the higher dosage is necessary.

THE "POTENCY RACE" is revealed with other statin medications, too. Baycol, the newest statin, was marketed in three sizes: 0.2 mg, 0.3, and 0.4 mg/day. Having three dosages was useful, but Bayer recommended the highest dosage for all patients initially. A dosage of 0.4 mg/day, which reduces LDL-C 34 percent, is certainly a reasonable dosage for some people, but so are the 0.3 mg and the 0.2 mg daily dosages, which reduce LDL-C 31 percent and 22 percent, respectively.

Moreover, individual response to Baycol can be highly variable. In a study published in the *American Journal of Cardiology*, 31 percent of people taking 0.3 mg/day of Baycol obtained 40-percent reductions in LDL-C.[43] Indeed, in one study, just 0.1 mg of Baycol reduced LDL-C by 30 percent in about a third of study subjects given this dose, and just 0.05 mg achieved the same desirable LDL-C reduction in 7 percent of subjects.[44] You may be one of these people, but if your doctor follows Bayer's dosage guidelines, you will receive 0.4 mg to start, as Bayer recommends.

Bayer now makes Baycol in a 0.8-mg dose, which some people need too. The point is that different people have different types of cholesterol problems and respond differently to statin drugs. This is why a wide range of doses is desirable, and why you and your physician should choose carefully in deciding where to start.

DOSAGE PROBLEMS WITH statin drugs aren't new. When Mevacor was introduced in 1987, the recommended initial dose was 20 mg/day. Soon, studies began appearing in which patients obtained excellent responses with half as much Mevacor.[45,46] In one of these studies, 24 of 28 patients achieved good results with a 50-percent-lower dose. The authors concluded: "Achievement of desirable values of cholesterol with 10 mg of lovastatin [Mevacor] was accompanied by less adverse effects and with significant financial saving. The calculated saving for lovastatin consumers in the USA could be an amount of $60,000,000."[47] Of course, Mevacor's price has risen over the last decade, so today the savings would be much greater.

George R. responded to low-dose Mevacor, but it wasn't his doctor's idea. George had suffered many medication reactions previously and thought it would be safer to start low. When his doctor prescribed the standard 20 mg/day of Mevacor, George broke the tablet into quarters. With this amount, his LDL-C dropped dramatically and he never needed a higher dose. People shouldn't have to make dosage decisions themselves, but neither should they be driven to do so by the imprecise methods of drug companies and doctors.

WHEN USED PROPERLY, Pravachol, Zocor, Lipitor, Mevacor, Lescol, and Baycol are excellent drugs. Statins have been proven not only to reduce cholesterol levels, but to reduce the incidence of heart attacks and coronary deaths. The enthusiasm of some doctors for these drugs is warranted—but not enough to warrant widespread overmedication and avoidable side effects. Multiple Web sites on the Internet attest to the devastating effects of these drugs in hundreds of people.

The pharmaceutical industry must curb the intense competition between statin manufacturers that has driven treatment toward higher, more potent initial doses and simplistic dosing regimens that cause avoidable side effects and increase long-term risks. Drug companies must provide dosage guidelines that differentiate between the needs of patients with and without coronary disease, and between patients with mild-to-moderate and severe cholesterol disorders. The pharmaceutical industry must provide prominent, highlighted guidelines that dosages should be chosen based on the amount of cholesterol lowering required by each person—which may sometimes require using dosages lower than generally recommended—and based on each person's individual characteristics and medical condition. Drug companies must remind physicians that people's responses to statin drugs vary greatly, and that the information on average reductions of cholesterol and LDL-C may not be a good indication of an individual's response.

The greatest problem with statin therapy has been getting patients into treatment and keeping them in treatment. To facilitate this, the medical profession and drug industry must work together to establish clear, medically sound parameters for initiating statin therapy with each patient as an individual. These guidelines should be placed prominently in package inserts and in the *PDR,* and the medication dosage recommendations should be consistent with these guidelines. The intense advertising for statin drugs should clarify that except for patients with cardiac disease, diabetes, or several risk factors, a healthy diet and exercise are the preferred initial treatment for most people with high cholesterol. Physicians and patients should be encouraged to remember that most people with elevated cholesterol have only mild-to-moderate elevations that do not require high-potency treatment initially.

Furthermore, patients' fears are not allayed when doctors ignore possible side effects. Dr. Gerald Glassman, Mercy Hospital's medical director of cardiology, said that many patients on statins may have side effects that doctors don't take the time to evaluate seriously. "A lot of patients complain of being weak and fatigued," he said. "We tend to discount unfairly many of the complaints elderly people have. Managed care wants us to give them the drug and let it be."[48]

The discovery of statin medications may be one of the pharmaceutical industry's greatest accomplishments. These drugs have allowed doctors to significantly reduce the risks of heart attacks and coronary deaths. However, competition among drug companies and overzealousness among physicians is producing avoidable problems with statin therapy, and a tide of concern is mounting. Balance needs to be established in the proper, individualized use of these very helpful drugs. Otherwise, the excesses that are occurring will increase, reports of severe side effects and deaths will become more common, and another promising group of drugs will become feared by the public.

One newswoman told me, "My elderly father was prescribed a drug for his high cholesterol, but he's afraid to take it." I hear this frequently. Perhaps this is one reason why, although 100 million Americans have elevated cholesterol levels and as many as 40 million require medication therapy, only a small percentage are in treatment.[49] And why so many who start treatment soon quit. Physicians may be enthusiastic about statins, but they should remember that many patients do not feel similar enthusiasm about having to take a costly prescription drug for the rest of their lives.

Applying the "Start low, go slow" approach to statin medications would allay many people's fears. Reducing cholesterol levels is not an emergency: There's time to properly measure the amount of cholesterol lowering required and even to perhaps start a little low just to test a person's response, because many people obtain greater LDL-C reductions than the mean. It is easy to gradually adjust the dosage upward, if necessary, until the correct amount is determined. This approach addresses people's concerns, it ensures that they do not receive any more medication than they require, and it avoids provoking unnecessary side effects—which is the first concern of most people starting new medications. It should likewise be the first concern of drug companies and doctors.

As this book was going to press, Baycol was withdrawn on August 8th, 2001. According to the FDA, this cholesterol-lowering drug was linked with 31 deaths from a severe form of muscle pain and degeneration called rhabdomyolysis, which is a dose-related reaction. At lower, safer doses, such reactions are less common, and if they do occur, they are usually less severe. The FDA reported that Baycol reactions occurred most often in the elderly. As we have seen, this group is often more sensitive to medications and more responsive to lower doses than younger adults. Yet Bayer's dosage recommendations for Baycol were the same for all adults (except for people with moderately severe liver or kidney disease).

TABLE 6.1

Mean LDL-C Reductions at Usual Initial Statin Doses

More is not necessarily better with medications. Using stronger drugs and dosages than required exposes people to unnecessary risks of side effects and potential long-term problems. Drugs and dosages should be gauged to the amount of cholesterol-lowering or LDL-C-lowering each person requires. Some people obtain even larger cholesterol reductions than the averages presented here.

Lipitor (atorvastatin)	10 mg	39%
Zocor (simvastatin)	20 mg	38%
Baycol (cerivastatin)	0.4 mg	34%
Pravachol (pravastatin)	20 mg	32%
Mevacor (lovastatin)	20 mg	27%
Lescol (fluvastatin)	40 mg	25%

Adapted from: Cohen, J.S. "Appropriate Initial Statin Doses for Primary Prevention Patients with Mild-to-Moderate Hypercholesterolemia." Submitted for publication, February 2001.

TABLE 6.2

Are You Being Overmedicated? Low, Proven-Effective Doses of Cholesterol-Lowering Medications

People exhibit wide variations in their blood concentrations and speed of drug elimination with statin drugs, indicating wide differences in their dosage requirements. These differences necessitate a range of dosages to fit people. Average reductions in LDL-C are listed, but individual response can vary greatly. Again, the drug and dosage should be individually matched to the specific amount of cholesterol-lowering or LDL-C–lowering required by each person.

Medication	Daily Dosage	*Average* Reduction in LDL-C**
Lipitor (atorvastatin)		
standard initial dosage:	10 mg	39%
effective lower dosages:	5 mg	28%
	2.5 mg	23%
Zocor (simvastatin)		
standard initial dosage:	20 mg	38%
effective lower dosages:	10 mg	30%
	5 mg	26%
Baycol (cerivastatin)		
standard initial dosage:	0.4 mg	34%
effective lower dosages:	0.3 mg	31%
	0.2 mg	22%
Pravachol (pravastatin)		
standard initial dosage:	20 mg	32%
effective lower dosage:	10 mg	22%
Mevacor (lovastatin)		
standard initial dosage:	20 mg	27%
effective lower dosage:	10 mg	21%
Lescol (fluvastatin)		
standard initial dosage:	40 mg	25%
effective lower dosage:	20 mg	22%

Adapted from: Cohen, J.S. "Appropriate Initial Statin Doses for Primary Prevention Patients with Mild-to-Moderate Hypercholesterolemia." Submitted for publication, February 2001.

This listing is for information purposes only. Readers should not change drugs or dosages unless specifically directed to do so by their own doctors.

TABLE 6.3

How Much Cholesterol Lowering Do You Actually Need?

Do You Have Any Risk Factors?

Risk factors include: Age (males 45 or more; females 55 or older); obesity; diabetes; hypertension; smoking; a family history of early coronary heart disease; or a high density lipoprotein-cholesterol (HDL-C, good cholesterol) level below 35. An HDL-C level above 60 offsets one risk factor.

Preferred Levels of Cholesterol

Total Cholesterol
<200	Desirable
200–239	Borderline High
240 or above	High

LDL Cholesterol*
<100	Optimal
100–129	Good
130–159	Borderline High
160–189	High
190 or above	Very High

HDL Cholesterol (Higher levels are desirable)
<40	Low
40–60	Good
60 or above	Optimal

*If you already have coronary or other atherosclerosis-related disease, or diabetes, an LDL-C above 100 is high.

PEOPLE NEEDING TREATMENT

Mild to Moderate Risk Group

Your risks of heart attacks and strokes are moderately increased if your LDL-C is:

With 0-1 risk factors: above 160.
With 2 or more risk factors: above 130.

High Risk Group

Your risks of heart attacks and strokes are greatly increased if your LDL-C is:

With 0-1 risk factors: above 190.
With 2 or more risk factors: above 160.

If you already have coronary or other atherosclerosis-related disease: above 100.

Adapted from: "Executive Summary of the Third Report of the National Cholesterol Education Program (NCEP) Expert Panel on Detection, Evaluation, and Treatment of High Blood Cholesterol in Adults." *JAMA*, 2001;285(19):2486–97.

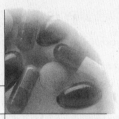

Why 50 to 75 Percent of People Quit Taking Their Medications for High Blood Pressure

CHOLESTEROL-LOWERING DRUGS aren't the only major medication group where dosages and side-effect rates are unnecessarily high. Antihypertensive drugs—for high blood pressure—cause even more side effects and drive as many patients from treatment.

Over 50 million people have hypertension (high blood pressure), but only 10 million currently receive adequate treatment. One issue has been to identify those with hypertension and have them receive treatment. An equally significant challenge is keeping them in treatment. Within a year of starting antihypertensive therapy, 50 percent of patients quit.[1-4]

"Hypertension remains one of the leading preventable causes of disability and death in the United States today," states a report by the Albert Einstein College Of Medicine. "Yet only 21% of patients with high blood pressure are under adequate therapeutic control. The statistics show that about half of treated hypertensive patients discontinue their therapy within a year."[5]

Hypertension is an insidious disease. It is a silent affliction that leads to kidney disease, heart disease, strokes, and other vascular disorders, drastically reducing longevity. Treatment is imperative. According to experts, if a 35-year-old man has a mildly elevated blood pressure of just 130/90, he will die four years earlier (on average) than an identical man without hypertension.[6] If the man's hypertension is 140/90, he will die nine years prematurely. If it's 150/100, he'll die seventeen years earlier, on average.

Hypertension accounts for more doctor visits in the United States than any other ailment; yet, almost as soon as people enter treatment, one half of them quit. One major reason is medication side effects that make people feel worse than before treatment. A person's quality of life can be greatly diminished by adverse effects such as dizziness, light-headedness, weakness, drowsiness, headache, fatigue, nausea, malaise, palpitations, confusion, swelling, muscle cramps, blurred vision, diarrhea, chronic cough, orthostatic hypotension (dizziness when standing up), or sexual dysfunctions. As an article in *Postgraduate Medicine* described it: "Often, the cure—the lowering of blood pressure—is perceived as being worse than the disease. . . . and when this is the case, the patient is unlikely to remain adherent and treatment may fail."[7]

As we have seen earlier, most side effects with antihypertensive drugs are dose-related—and therefore avoidable. Individual sensitivities to antihypertensive drugs are widely recognized, and most authorities on hypertension subscribe to the "Start low, go slow" approach. When people are medicated carefully, they usually do well on these medications.

"I always individualize treatment," one expert told me. "This improves accuracy, and patients like it better. Some patients have been to so many doctors and had so many side effects, they become sensitized. They almost demand lower doses. That's not a bad idea anyway, because if people are overmedicated, their blood pressures can really drop, which has its own dangers. Taking time for a detailed medication history and starting medications low almost always works."

A 1999 article similarly explained, "Unless acute target organ in-volvement [such as kidney damage or heart failure] is already present, there are no compelling reasons to lower blood pressure quickly. In-stead, beginning with relatively low doses of medications and slowly bringing the blood pressure to goal helps avoid troublesome medica-tion side effects."[8]

Going easy has other advantages. It allows people to make further adjustments that are known to reduce high blood pressure—to im-prove their diets, reduce salt intake, lose weight, initiate exercise, and undertake stress reduction or meditation. Sometimes these adjust-ments allow people to avoid medication treatment altogether, or to respond to lower medication doses and thereby minimize side effects.[9]

When Hal developed hypertension, his doctor prescribed Capoten at an initial dosage of 12.5 mg/day—substantially less than the 50 to 75 mg/day recommended by the manufacturer. At his doctor's sug-gestion, Hal also reduced his work stress and began meditating. His blood pressure stabilized, and a higher dosage was never needed. I contacted Hal's physician and asked about his approach.

"My philosophy's real, real simple," he explained. "I give just enough to make it work. I usually start by underdosing people. If hy-pertension isn't horrific, and if you 'crawl up' with the dosage, you avoid scaring people by overshooting and making them feel bad. Very often, their blood vessels relax over a period of time and you wind up ultimately needing less medication."

UNFORTUNATELY, MANY DOCTORS don't take the time (or the insurers don't allow them the time) to tailor medication doses to pa-tients. Instead, they rely on drug company information, but as we have seen with many other drugs, drug company information can be in-complete or outdated. Package inserts, the *PDR*, and drug-company advertising often omit information about the lowest, safest drug doses. This is a particularly serious problem with antihypertensive drugs.

The information gap is so large that in March 2001, I published an article in the *Archives of Internal Medicine*[10] comparing the initial doses of antihypertensive drugs recommended by the drug companies with the dosages recommended by the foremost panel of experts in America, the Joint National Committee on the Detection, Evaluation, and Treatment of High Blood Pressure (JNC). The JNC convenes every five years and publishes an updated report on the status of antihypertensive therapy and recommendations regarding all phases of hypertension treatment.[11] The results of my analysis were astonishing.

Of 40 antihypertensive drugs, the experts recommended substantially lower initial doses for 23 drugs—that's 58 percent of the major antihypertensive drugs. (See Table 7.1.) In other words, if you receive one of these 23 drugs from a doctor relying on drug-company guidelines, your chances of getting overmedicated will be greatly increased. With 22 of the 23 drugs, the drug company initial doses were at least 100 percent higher than the experts' preferred doses. Obviously the problem isn't just a few antihypertensive drugs, but the majority of them.

Moreover, these unnecessarily high initial doses occurred with some of our newest and most prescribed antihypertensive medications. Among them was Norvasc, the seventh most prescribed drug in America in 1999, for which patients filled 27 million prescriptions and spent $1.4 billion. Pfizer's recommended initial dose of Norvasc for most patients is 5 mg/day—100 percent higher than the 2.5 mg the JNC suggests. Patients also paid for 38 million prescriptions for atenolol (Tenormin) in 1999. The JNC recommends starting this drug at 25 mg daily. Originally the manufacturer recommended 100 mg—400 percent more medicine. Finally, decades later, it reduced its recommended dose to 50 mg, still 100 percent more than the experts suggest.

The problem involves other top-sellers, including Zestril, Prinivil, Altace, Inderal (propranolol), Cardura, Cozaar. Getting the very lowest initial doses is especially important with antihypertensive drugs because, as an older specialist told me, "With blood pressure, it's easy to overshoot the mark. When we give normal doses, we spend the rest of our lives combating side effects."

Wendy C.'s experience is typical. Wendy reacted to one antihypertensive drug after another, failing treatment four times. Her side effects were entirely dose-related, usually occurring with the first doses, a sure sign of overmedication. Wendy was motivated. She knew her hypertension posed a serious threat. Several relatives had died prematurely from hypertension-related heart attacks and strokes. Wendy wanted to get her hypertension under control, but her repeated problems with medications made her feel hopeless.

"I don't know what I'm going to do," Wendy told me. "I'm so sensitive, I can't even tolerate the lowest dose of some medications."

But if the lowest doses recommended by the drug companies and prescribed by doctors are really the lowest, least side-effect-prone dosages, cases like Wendy's aren't so mysterious.

Starting with the very lowest, safest, antihypertensive drug dosages is the key to successful treatment; yet, most physicians still rely on drug company information to guide them. More than 90 percent of physicians turn to the *PDR* for dosage information,[12,13] whereas a survey revealed that many physicians have never heard of the JNC or its low-dose guidelines.[14]

The dosage problem is compounded when people require increases in their dosages. Drug companies usually recommend jumps in dosage of 100 percent. For example, Hytrin is recommended at 1, 2, 5, and 10 mg; Norvasc at 2.5, 5, and 10 mg. But some people's bodies aren't prepared for or simply don't need 100-percent increases in dosage, and the result is dose-related side effects. The smallest jump recommended by drug companies is usually 50 percent, but even this amount is excessive for many people. With methods like these, it is no surprise that most medication side effects occur either when people start new medications or when the dosage is increased.

The fact that many of these dosage discrepancies occur with newer medications indicates that these problems have not been rectified by the drug companies or the FDA. Worse, although it is widely accepted that older people often are very sensitive to the effects of antihypertensive drugs and should be started with even lower doses than prescribed to younger individuals, with 37 of the 45 (82 percent) of the top-selling antihypertensive drugs, the drug companies don't even bother to recommend lower initial doses for seniors. Indeed, in their advertising in medical journals, some drug companies boast that doctors can prescribe the very same starting doses to all patients, including very old patients taking multiple medications. Perhaps this makes good advertising, but it doesn't make good treatment.

THE CONSEQUENCES OF such methods are evident with hydrochlorothiazide (HCTZ), a popular diuretic for treating hypertension and a perennial top-selling drug. For decades, drug companies recommended initial dosages of 25, 50, and even 100 mg of HCTZ (as Hydrodiuril, Esidrix, and Oretic) per day. After many years, the highest of these dosages were dropped, and in 2000 Merck recommended 25 mg/day for starting treatment with Hydrodiuril. Meanwhile, for many years experts have been recommending only 12.5 mg of HCTZ and sometimes just 6.25 mg, one half to one sixteenth of the original drug-company doses.

I asked a nationally recognized hypertension expert at the University of California, San Diego, about this. "It has been obvious for many years that standard doses of HCTZ for hypertension are much too large," he replied. "As I review many older studies, it appears that very low-dose diuretic therapy decreased the incidence of heart attack and sudden cardiac death, while moderate size doses provided no cardiac protection, and larger doses harm people."

Unrecognized problems have occurred with other antihypertensive drugs. With ACE inhibitors, far more people develop chronic coughs than the drug companies' research suggested. For example, according to Merck, the frequency of coughing due to Vasotec is 2.2 percent, but in a 1989 study in the *Archives of Internal Medicine,* 11 percent of the patients quit treatment because of a persistent, dry, severe cough, and many other patients who stayed in treatment also complained of coughs.[15] The problem was so pervasive that a 1996 article in the *European Journal of Clinical Pharmacology* was aptly titled "ACE-Inhibitor-Induced Cough, An Adverse Drug Reaction Unrecognized for Several Years."[16]

A 1997 article in the *Journal of the American Geriatrics Society* reported changes in brain structure and diminished performance in cognitive testing among patients using calcium channel blockers and loop diuretics.[17] An accompanying editorial advised caution in interpreting these preliminary results,[18] and further investigation is under way. Meanwhile, in 2000, the use of calcium channel blockers for treating hypertension became even more suspect following a report that although these drugs do lower blood pressure, they may not prevent heart attacks or heart failure as well as other antihypertensive drugs.[19] Suddenly, experts were recommending that calcium channel blockers such as Norvasc, Cardizem, and Procardia, frequent favorites of physicians, should no longer be considered first-line drugs for hypertension.[20]

Similarly, more than twenty-five years after Motrin was introduced, it was finally recognized that the use of Motrin or other anti-inflammatory drugs may counter the effects of antihypertensive drugs such as HCTZ.[21] Indeed, anti-inflammatory drugs may actually increase the likelihood of developing hypertension in older people.[22]

The discovery of new side effects only after many years of use in the general population is not unique to antihypertensive drugs. This occurs with medications of all types. Because hypertension must be treated, the best protection is to employ the lowest, safest dosage that each person requires. Again, this can only be accomplished by starting low and, if necessary, increasing gradually. Many people display sensitivities when new chemicals are introduced to their systems, but with repeated exposure, most sensitivities recede as people's bodies adjust. It's the same with antihypertensive medications—and most medications.

Sometimes severe hypertension is an emergency and requires immediate, full-dosage treatment. But most situations don't require such intensive therapy initially, and most people ultimately do much better if allowed to adjust to antihypertensive medications gradually and safely. Unfortunately, often this is not reflected in how drug companies develop and market antihypertensive drugs or in how doctors prescribe them.

TABLE 7.1

Recommended Initial Dosages for Antihypertensive Drugs: Drug Companies Versus the Joint National Committee on Hypertension

For initiating treatment in adults with mild-to-moderate hypertension.

Medication	Drug Company Daily Dosages	JNC Daily Dosages
ACE Inhibitors (discrepancies with 4 of 8 drugs in this group)		
Accupril (quinapril):	10 mg	5 mg
Altace (ramipril):	2.5 mg	1.25 mg
Capoten (captopril):	50-75 mg	25 mg
Prinivil, Zestril (lisinopril):	10 mg	5 mg
Angiotensin II Receptor Blockers (discrepancies with 1 of 2 drugs in this group; 1 drug not testable**)		
Cozaar (losartan):	50 mg	25 mg
Beta Blockers (discrepancies with 6 of 10 drugs)		
Inderal (propranolol):	80 mg	40 mg
Kerlone (betaxolol):	10 mg	5 mg
Levatol (penbutolol):	20 mg	10 mg
Lopressor (metoprolol):	100 mg	50 mg
Sectral (acebutolol):	400 mg	200 mg
Tenormin (atenolol):	50 mg	25 mg***
Zebeta (bisoprolol):	5 mg	2.5 mg*
Calcium Antagonists (discrepancies with 4 of 5 drugs in this group, 1 not testable**)		
Calan, Isoptin, Verelan (verapamil):	120-180 mg	90 mg
Cardizem, Dilacor (diltiazem):	180-240 mg	120 mg
Norvasc (amlodipine):	5 mg	2.5 mg
Plendil (felodipine):	5 mg	2.5 mg
Diuretics (discrepancies with 7 of 9 drugs in this group)		
Demadex (torsemide):	10 mg	5 mg
Edecrin (ethacrynic acid):	50 mg	25 mg
HCTZ (hydrochlorothiazide):	25 mg	12.5 mg
Lasix (furosemide):	80 mg	40 mg
Spironolactone:	50 mg	25 mg
Thalitone (chlorthalidone):	15 mg	12.5 mg
Triamterene:	25 mg	200 mg

*The *PDR*'s "usual" initial dosage of Zebeta is 5 mg/day, but it then adds that 2.5 mg may be sufficient for "some patients." Experts recommend 2.5 mg initially for all patients.

**Five drugs are produced as capsules, coated or irregularly-shaped pills that cannot be prescribed at doses lower than recommended by the *PDR*.

***The *PDR*'s usual initial dose of Norvase is 5 mg/day, but the *PDR* adds that 2.5 mg/day may be sufficient for small, elderly, or debilitated patients. The *JNC* recommends 2.5 mg initially for all patients.

116

This listing is for information purposes only. Readers should not change drugs or dosages unless specifically directed to do so by their own doctors.

Adapted from: Cohen, J.S. "Adverse Drug Effects, Compliance, and the Initial Doses of Antihypertensive Drugs Recommended by the Joint National Committee (JNC) vs. the Physicians' Desk Reference. *Archives of Internal Medicine,* 2001;161:880-85.

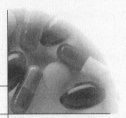

Chapter 8

Why Seniors Are at the Greatest Risk

THE HIGH INCIDENCE of side effects impacts the elderly more than any other group. Although people over age 60 constitute about 19 percent of the population, they account for 39 percent of all hospitalizations and 51 percent of all deaths related to medication reactions. Indeed, 10 to 17 percent of all hospitalizations for seniors are related to side effects, and once they are hospitalized, the elderly run the greatest risk of a major medication reaction or medication-related death. Many of these side effects occur at standard medication doses, as an article in *The Journal of the American Board of Family Practice* reported, "Nine percent of our elderly patients' hospital admissions were caused by adverse reactions that were due to usual doses of medications commonly prescribed for elderly patients."[1]

These statistics are alarming enough, but they may be underestimates. As *The New England Journal of Medicine* reported: "The overall incidence of adverse drugs reactions in the elderly is two to three times that found in young adults. Furthermore, the incidence is probably underestimated, because adverse drug reactions are less readily recognized by the elderly themselves and because the reactions may mimic the characteristics of disease states."[2]

The elderly are more prone to side effects for several reasons. Their bodies process medications more slowly than younger people, causing blood concentrations of medications to reach higher levels and take longer to be eliminated. Seniors' tissues may also be more sensitive to the impact of drugs. These and other factors are why older people require the most cautious, individualized usage of medications. As we've seen, however, drug companies don't develop drugs to be individualized. Drug companies and doctors prefer expedient, easy-to-use methods that disregard people's individual differences and trigger unnecessary side effects in millions each year. Among these millions, seniors rank first.

This is why many experts in geriatrics recommend that older patients should be prescribed doses substantially lower than those prescribed to younger patients, at least initially. A 1990 article in the medical journal *Drug Safety* stated: "Starting doses can often be reduced in the elderly, and clinical and therapeutic monitoring of effect is mandatory."[3] A journal article titled "How not to poison your elderly patients" put it another way: ". . . [T]he starting dose [for older people] should be lower than that recommended for younger adults; stepwise adjustment should be made until optimal therapeutic response is obtained; the maximum tolerated dose may well be lower than for younger individuals."[4] Public Citizen's book *Worst Pills, Best Pills II* adds: "If drug therapy is indicated, in most cases it is safer to start with the dose which is lower than the usual adult dose."[5]

Using lower doses for older people not only is common sense, it also makes medical sense. According to a 1999 article in the *Journal of the American Geriatrics Society*, "Choosing the correct dose of a drug therapy is critical when prescribing for older people because adverse effects are often dose-related. The conventional wisdom has been to 'start low and go slow.' "[6] Yet, the drug companies don't even bother to recommend lower doses for older people with many of our most popular medications. In Table 8.1 (page 127), which I published in *Geriatrics* in February 2000, I list eighty-six top-selling drugs for which drug companies tell doctors to prescribe *the very same initial doses to older and younger people.* Let's take a look at a few of these drugs, which represent some of today's most prescribed groups of medications.

Antihistamines

Allegra

If you are 65 or older and if your doctor prescribes you the antihistamine Allegra, the dose will likely be 60 mg twice a day, because this is the only dosage that Hoechst Marion Roussel recommends (except for people with kidney disease). Allegra is essentially one-size-fits-all, so your age, weight, state of health, or use of other medications do not affect the recommended dosage. Nor does it matter that the blood concentration of Allegra rises 99 percent higher in seniors than in younger adults. Elevated blood concentrations mean increased potency and increased risks of side effects and drug interactions, so a lower dose for older adults would make obvious sense, especially since a lower dose of Allegra was proven effective.[7] But if your doctor wants to try a lower dose, Hoechst Marion Roussel doesn't make it easy: Allegra comes in only one size, 60 mg, and only as a capsule.

Hoechst Marion Roussel also produced Seldane, which was withdrawn in 1997 because it provoked cardiac arrhythmias and deaths. Seldane was also an antihistamine and a one-size-fits-all drug. A substantially lower dose had been proven effective, but it was never developed.[8,9]

Claritin

Claritin is America's top-selling antihistamine and the ninth topselling drug overall in 1999. Like Allegra, Claritin is essentially one-size-fits-all. In fact, Claritin's dosing goes a step further than Allegra's. With Claritin, Schering recommends the same dose (except for people with liver or kidney dysfunction) not only for Shaquille

O'Neal and Ally McBeal, and not only for 90-year-old seniors, but even for 6-year-old children.

However, in its information in the *PDR*, Schering acknowledges that Claritin blood levels rise 50 percent higher and last far longer in older people. This means greater risks of side effects and drug interactions. It also means that many seniors need less Claritin. This is borne out by several people I know who experienced side effects at Claritin's standard dose but who have done quite nicely by splitting the Claritin tablet.

Medications for Ulcers, Gastritis, and Esophagitis

Prilosec

From 1997–2000, Prilosec was the top-selling drug in America. In 1999, Prilosec was prescribed 31,886,000 times and earned a single-drug sales record of $4,187,000,000 for AstraZeneca. The usual starting dose of Prilosec is 20 mg/day for all adults, including the elderly. Yet, according to AstraZeneca's studies in *healthy* seniors, Prilosec rises 40 to 50 percent higher and lasts nearly 50 percent longer in the bloodstream. These increases are likely much higher in older people with other illnesses or taking other medications, further increasing their risks, but AstraZeneca provides no information about this in the package insert or *PDR*.

There is ample evidence that a lower dose of Prilosec may suffice for many seniors. Several studies have demonstrated the effectiveness of one-half doses of Prilosec.[10,11] Unfortunately, this information was published in little-known journals, and AstraZeneca has never added it to the Prilosec package insert or *PDR* write-up, so few doctors know about the effectiveness of low-dose Prilosec.

That's not all. If you are older and Asian-American, your risks with Prilosec may be multiplied. AstraZeneca acknowledges that Prilosec blood levels increase "approximately four-fold . . . in Asian subjects compared to Caucasians." If the blood concentration rises 400 percent higher in Asian-Americans of average age, how much further does it rise in elderly Asian-Americans? AstraZeneca does suggest "dose adjustments" for Asian-Americans, but this sound advice is buried amid columns of information in the package insert's "Clinical Pharmacology" section, which most doctors don't read. Yet, in the insert's "Dosage and Administration" section, where doctors check for this type of information, AstraZeneca doesn't mention dose adjustments for Asian-Americans at all.

Zantac, Axid, Pepcid, Tagamet

For decades, doctors prescribed these drugs more than any others for ulcers, gastritis, and esophagitis. Many times, Zantac was the top-selling drug in America. Lower doses of these drugs worked,[12-20] but most doctors didn't know it, so doctors prescribed full doses to people with mild conditions that today are handled by low-dose, over-the-counter versions of these same drugs. In the case of Zantac, the package insert did inform doctors that although Zantac's recommended dose was 150 mg twice daily, a dose of 100 mg twice daily was just as effective—and yet, I never met a doctor or pharmacist who ever noticed this information in the package insert or *PDR*.

Cholesterol-Lowering Drugs

The Statins: Lipitor, Zocor, Mevacor, Pravachol, Baycol, Lescol

In Chapter 6, I described many of the problems with this top-selling group of drugs. Here, I'll just mention that although Pfizer recommends the same 10-mg starting dose of Lipitor for everyone, Lipitor blood levels rise 40 percent higher and last much longer in seniors. This is an indication of the usefulness of lower doses with this population, and it explains why the majority of the many complaints I receive about Lipitor come from older people. But Pfizer doesn't make a lower-dose Lipitor pill. Other statins—Pravachol, Lescol—are recommended at milder initial doses. Zocor, Mevacor, and Baycol are produced in low-dose pills, and their manufacturers provide doctors with information about the effectiveness of these lower doses. But Lipitor is easy to use, and it is the top-selling cholesterol-lowering drug in America.

Antihypertensive Drugs

As discussed in Chapter 7, antihypertensive drugs constitute perhaps the most prescribed and one of the most side-effect-prone groups of drugs in America. Side effects such as tiredness, dizziness, sexual dysfunctions, and others are frequent, and they diminish patients' quality of life and cause many to quit treatment. Within one year of starting antihypertensive medication, 16 to 50 percent quit treatment.[21–24]

Seniors are most likely to need antihypertensive drugs and to be most vulnerable to their side effects. Knowing this, virtually every medical authority recommends starting seniors at very low doses of antihypertensive drugs. Yet, with 37 of the 44 best-selling antihypertensive drugs, the drug companies tell doctors to initiate treatment at the very same doses for seniors as for younger adults. (See Table 8.1, page 127.)

It isn't as if we lack scientific data about the greater risks of these drugs in older people. For example, we know that the antihypertensive drug Zestril, America's seventeenth most prescribed drug in 1999, rises to 100 percent higher blood levels in seniors. Nonetheless, the manufacturer's recommended initial dose is the same for seniors as for young adults. This makes no sense medically. Zestril isn't the only antihypertensive drug marketed this way. Similar problems exist with many of these medications.

Obtaining proper, side-effect-free treatment for hypertension is extremely important for older people. Hypertension is a common cause of heart attacks and strokes, and it can cause losses in cognitive abilities such as thinking and remembering.[25]

Anti-inflammatory Drugs

Celebrex

Each year for more than a decade, more than 41,000 seniors have been hospitalized because of adverse reactions associated with anti-inflammatory drugs such as Motrin, Orudis, Naprosyn, and over a dozen others.[26] More than 3,300 seniors died annually just from gastrointestinal hemorrhages with these drugs.[27] The newer anti-inflammatories, Vioxx and Celebrex, seem safer in this regard, but they also have been linked to ulcers and bleeding as well as kidney damage and other serious side effects. Because of the well-documented dangers of anti-inflammatory drugs, the FDA requires all drug companies to place statements in their package inserts about the importance of using the lowest effective doses of these drugs with each patient. But do the drug companies' policies really make it possible to use the lowest effective dose?

In chapter 2, I described how millions of people are overmedicated with anti-inflammatory drugs and how drug companies have failed to provide low-dose information to doctors and patients. With the record-breaking new anti-inflammatory drug Celebrex, drug-company methodology isn't much better, especially in regard to older people. In the Celebrex package insert, Searle notes that "the incidence of adverse experiences tended to be higher in elderly patients." It also states that seniors develop 40 to 50 percent higher blood levels of Celebrex—and higher blood levels are directly linked to higher risks of side effects. Yet, Searle doesn't recommend lower doses of Celebrex for seniors.

Searle does specifically recommend that, with seniors, doctors should "initiate therapy at the lowest recommended dose." But this is ludicrous, because there is no "lowest recommended dose" for Celebrex's most common usage, osteoarthritis (the arthritis of aging). The recommended dose is a one-size-fits-all 100 mg twice daily. Everyone from the 25-year-old football player with a bad knee to the 85-year-old woman with osteoarthritis and four other maladies gets 100 mg of Celebrex twice daily. And even though it is now known that a 50-percent lower dose of Celebrex—50 mg twice daily—is effective,[28] this dosage is difficult to use because Celebrex comes only in 100- and 200-mg capsules.

The result is predictable. Beginning with her first dose of Celebrex, Jill R., age 64, suffered, in her own words, "increased blood pressure, heart rate too slow and irregular, crying at the drop of a hat for no reason, irritable and impatient with all around me, feeling very drugged, inability to focus either visually or mentally." Such side effects are typically dose-related and might have been avoided by starting with a lower dose. But how was Jill's doctor to know about low-dose Celebrex? As we have seen with other drugs, the Celebrex package insert and *PDR* description mention nothing about a lower, safer, proven-effective Celebrex dosage.

IT WOULD BE comforting if most of these problems occurred with older drugs, and that with newer drugs the pharmaceutical industry was producing more flexible, individualized doses, especially for seniors. But Celebrex was introduced in 1999, and Lipitor in 1997. Prilosec was approved in the early 1990's, and Claritin and Allegra represent the newest generation of antihistamines. I see ads each month for newly introduced medications, and many of them are offered at identical doses for older and younger patients, which the advertising extols. Obviously the new FDA regulations for protecting the elderly leave a lot to be desired. Perhaps it's because, as recent analyses have shown, older patients are still not adequately represented in new drug studies.

Why aren't dosages designed for seniors? We have long known about seniors' heightened sensitivities and heightened risks with medications. Decades ago, medical science recognized that seniors' diminished liver and kidney functioning caused them to process and eliminate medications more slowly than younger people. In addition, most seniors have other illnesses, and 78 percent of seniors take at least one prescription drug and 60 percent take at least one nonprescription remedy.[29,30] The average older person takes three drugs—prescription and nonprescription—on a daily basis.[31] All of these factors translate into markedly greater risks of side effects and drug interactions—the risks of which are increased if the doses are unnecessarily high.

To this, add the unending revelations of newly identified side effects with widely used drugs. For example, a 2000 study in the *Archives of Internal Medicine* linked anti-inflammatory drugs with congestive heart failure in older people.[32] Even though anti-inflammatory drugs have been used for a quarter century, this complication—which may be as massive in scope as anti-inflammatory drugs' provocation of ulcers and intestinal bleeding—was never evident. Why? Heart failure is so common in older people, and the use of multiple medications makes identifying a particular cause so difficult, that the association between anti-inflammatory drugs and heart failure was never clear. However, the authors of this study were convinced: "The burden of illness resulting from anti-inflammatory drug-related congestive heart failure may exceed that from gastrointestinal tract damage. Anti-inflammatory drugs should be used with caution in patients with a history of cardiovascular disease."[33]

These types of oversights occur all the time. In a *New York Times* News Service interview, Dr. Steffi Woolhandler, of the Harvard Medical School, stated: "A lot of the problem is that doctors frequently ascribe side effects of drugs to old age. . . . If a patient loses memory or loses balance, they say it's old age."[34] Thus, a lot of problems aren't discovered until years later—years after many people, especially older people, have been harmed. Other medication problems aren't discovered at all and continue to cause harm.

All of these factors explain why *uncertainty is always a major part of the equation with any medication in seniors.* Or, as a 1991 journal article put it: "The main problem of the elderly is the unpredictability of their response to drugs."[35] This is why it is so important to "Start low, go slow" with all medications, especially with older people, making sure that the very lowest amount of medication necessary is used initially.

But as we have seen, the drug companies often recommend quite the opposite. Moreover, for seniors who require higher doses, drug companies often suggest dose increases of 100 percent. This is *not* gradual dosing. Thus, side effects are frequently triggered when doctors increase doses by jumps that are too large for many seniors' needs or tolerance. Premarin, Prilosec, Lipitor, Zocor, Zoloft, Prevacid, Claritin, and Norvasc are all ranked among the ten top-selling drugs in America—and, like many other drugs, all of them are started at the very same doses for older and younger people alike. When increases in doses are required, the drugs are increased in 100-percent jumps for older and younger people alike.

Some doctors recognize the absurdity of this and use their own better judgment. "I use less of everything," one internist told me. "For very old people, I use doses that are so low, they border on the homeopathic—but they work."

Such methods prevent side effects. Indeed, a 2000 study of nursing home patients found that of the 20,000 fatal or life-threatening medication reactions occurring each year, "80% are preventable."[36] Many older people know about the threat of overmedication. That's why safety is their first concern with medication treatment. Millions of seniors attempt to alter their doses themselves, trying to avoid or reduce side effects. But people altering their own medications is dangerous, because the dosage may be too low, making people vulnerable to major illness, and this isn't going to solve the overall problem.

Seniors are said to be our most vocal political group, but they have been silent about the risks they face and the damage they suffer from improper drug company policies. We hear a lot about seniors' difficulties in paying for prescription drugs: Their outrage is justified. But overmedication is a bigger and costlier problem, and it has yet to be brought into the light. Not only does flexible dosing that fits patients reduce side effects, but using lower doses can reduce prescription costs as well.

Seniors' groups and associations must examine these issues and demand change. The drug companies have made it clear that they aren't going to improve their methods willingly. Doctors either don't have the data or do not bother to use it. The demand for change will have to come from seniors, who are paying the costs in money and in side effects for the widespread overmedication that drug company policies perpetuate.

TABLE 8.1

Eighty-Six Top-Selling Medications for Which Drug Companies Do Not Provide Lower Initial Doses for Older Patients

Experts in geriatrics recommend lower medication doses for older people, but drug companies frequently ignore this scientifically sound advice. Thus, with these medications, seniors are started at the very same doses as 25-year-olds.

- **Antidepressants:** Celexa (citalopram), Desyrel (trazodone), Effexor and Effexor XR (venlafaxine), Remeron (mirtazapine), Serzone (nefazodone), Sinequan (doxepin), Wellbutrin (bupropion), Wellbutrin RX (bupropion), Zoloft (sertraline).
- **Anti-inflammatories:** Anaprox, Anaprox DS, Naprelan, Naprosyn, EC-Naprosyn (naproxen), Celebrex (celecoxib), Clinocil (sulindac), Daypro (oxaprozin), Feldene (piroxicam), Indocin (indomethacin), Motrin (ibuprofen), Relafen (nabumetone), Vioxx (rofecoxib), Voltaren (diclofenac).
- **Antihistamines:** Allegra (fexofenadine), Claritin (loratadine), Zyrtec (cetirizine).
- **Antihypertensives:** Accupril (quinapril), Aceon (perindopril), Aldactone (spironolactone), Aldomet (methyldopa), Altace (ramipril), Atacand (candesartan), Avapro (irbesartan), Blocadren (timolol), Capoten (captopril), Cardizem (diltiazem), Cardura (doxazosin), Catrol (carteolol), Coreg (carvedilol), Cozaar (losartan), Demadex (torsemide), Diovan (valsartan), Dyrenium (triamterene), Edecrin (ethacrynic acid), Hydrodiuril (hydrochlorothiazide, HCTZ), Hytrin (terazosin), Inderal (propranolol), Lasix (furosemide), Levatol (penbutolol), Lopressor (metoprolol), Mavik (trandolapril), Micardis (telmisartan), Midamor (amiloride), Minipress (prazosin), Monopril (fosinopril), Mykrox (metolazone), Nadolol, Prinivil (lisinopril),* Procardia (nifedipine), Sectral (acebutolol), Sular (nisoldipine), Tenex (guanfacine), Teveten (eprosatan), Thalitone (chlorthalidone), Tiazac (diltiazem), Trandate (labetolol), Univasc (moexipril), Vasotec (enalapril), Zebeta (bisoprolol), Zestril (lisinopril).*
- **Cholesterol-Lowering:** Baycol (cerivastatin), Lescol (fluvastatin), Lipitor (atorvastatin), Mevacor (lovastatin), Zocor (simvastatin).

128

- **For Ulcers/Gastritis/Esophagitis:** Axid (nizatidine), Pepcid (famotidine), Prevacid (lansoprazole), Prilosec (omeprazole), Tagamet (cimetidine), Zantac (ranitidine).
- **Others:** Cytotec (misoprostol), Enbrel (colchicine, etanercept), Lopid (gemfibrozil), Propecia (finasteride), Transderm-Scop (scopolamine), Xenical (orlistat), Zofran (ondansetron), Zyban (bupropion), Zyloprim (allopurinol).

*Advises more careful dose adjustments, when necessary, for older patients.

This listing is for information purposes only. Readers should not change drugs or dosages unless specifically directed to do so by their own doctors.

Adapted from: Cohen, J.S. "Adverse Drug Reactions: Effective Low-Dose Therapies for Older Patients." *Geriatrics,* Feb. 2000; 55(2):54–64.

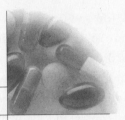

Chapter 9

How the Drug Companies Slant Drug Research, Limit Information to Doctors and Consumers, and Secure High Profits

UP TO THIS POINT, we have examined how drug-company policies result in the following problems:

- recommended dosages exceeding the needs of patients
- huge deficiencies in the dosage information provided to physicians and consumers
- questionable statistics on side effects
- years or decades of delay in discovering serious side effects with top-selling drugs
- failure to correct dosage or side-effect information after errors have been discovered
- inattention to the needs of different populations, such as women and older patients
- inattention to the basic scientific principle of individual variation in response to drugs.

Now we will examine the question of how these problems are perpetuated and why they are so difficult to change. This chapter will describe the influence that drug companies exert over medical research, the FDA, physicians, and patients. Moreover, we will see how drug companies not only control both the development and dosaging of medications, but also by controlling the main sources of drug information, how medications are perceived and understood by doctors and consumers. Ultimately this level of drug-company influence maintains a status quo in which millions of dose-related side effects and thousands of deaths continue to occur each year—with scant notice by the media or the public.

Drug-Company Influences on Research

Drug companies conduct virtually all of the early research on new drugs. Dosage studies, which are held during the earliest phase of human testing, are typically just a few weeks or months in length. These studies are conducted on a few dozen to a few hundred carefully selected subjects, although the drug may ultimately be prescribed to millions. New drug studies often focus on one type of usage, even though a drug may be used for a dozen other conditions for which it was never tested. The result, as Dr. Carl Peck stated in *The Journal of Clinical Pharmacology:* "Often, a commercial sponsor does not want [the earliest phases of research] to be prolonged, and hence, the extra time needed to explore the full dose range and various dose intervals to obtain good dose and concentration information may not be committed. . . . On too many occasions, failure to define dose-concentration-response relationships leads to unacceptable toxicity or adverse effect rates, marginal evidence of effectiveness, and a lack of information on how to individualize dosing."[1]

Later phases of new drug research are intended to confirm a new drug's efficacy and to ensure its safety. These phases are larger and longer, and they are supposed to be conducted scientifically and without bias. But by underwriting most of these studies, the drug companies wield enormous influence—influence so pervasive that in May

2000, Dr. Marcia Angell, the editor in chief of *The New England Journal of Medicine,* published an article titled "Is Academic Medicine for Sale?"

Academic medical institutions such as medical schools and teaching hospitals have traditionally conducted most studies of new drugs. Because of high ethical standards and independence from drug-company influence, the quality of information from academic medical research has always been considered high. Unfortunately, this is changing, Dr. Angell said, as "academic medical institutions are themselves growing increasingly beholden to industry."

This presents many dangers, Dr. Angell warned, for the integrity of doctors and for the safety of patients:

> One obvious concern is that these ties will bias research. . . . Researchers might undertake studies on the basis of whether they can get industry funding, not whether the studies are scientifically important. . . . It would skew research toward finding trivial differences between drugs, because these differences can be exploited for marketing.[2]

Dr. Angell described how drug companies use financial support to gain leverage over how research projects are conducted. Marketing objectives supersede true medical inquiry. "When the boundaries between industry and academic medicine become as blurred as they now are, the business goals of industry influence the mission of medical schools. . . ." Medical centers are becoming "outposts for industry" where "faculty and medical students essentially carry out industry research." New physicians, interns, residents, and students learn in environments with an "overemphasis on drugs and devices. . . . As the critics of medicine so often charge, young physicians learn that for every problem, there is a pill (and a drug company representative to explain it)."[3]

Drug-company money represents "a Faustian bargain" for medical institutions, Dr. Angell wrote, because drug companies can play one institution against the next, ultimately selecting the one most willing to weaken its ethical standards to fulfill drug-company interests. Over time, any medical institution wishing to survive will have to compromise its values and bow to drug-company preferences. Dr. Angell warned that "academic institutions and their clinical faculty members must take care not to be open to the charge that they are for sale."[4]

These warnings may have come too late. Dr. Angell herself described how difficult it was to find an independent expert to review an article about a new psychiatric drug, because every expert she asked had financial arrangements with the drug companies.[5] A heart researcher at the University of California, San Diego, echoed these concerns: "Our group is trying to conduct research without drug company money, which presents a lot of complications and limitations for us. We are the only ones I know doing this."

Indeed, rather than avoid conflicts of interests with drug companies, financially strapped medical centers today seek faculty members with drug-company connections. "Many academic centers now require researchers to "justify" their salaries—i.e., obtain research money," Dr. Jonathan Leibowitz, of the University of Pittsburgh Medical Center, wrote in response to Dr. Angell's article. This has been made worse by reductions in insurance reimbursements and "the new, corporate mentality that now pervades medicine." Leibowitz added that it is unrealistic to expect academic centers to restrict these relationships, "especially when many of these institutions are actively recruiting faculty members to run for-profit clinical trials sponsored by the pharmaceutical industry."[6]

Lainie Friedman Ross, M.D., Ph.D., of the University of Chicago, also replied in *The New England Journal of Medicine:* "Dr. Angell is right to acknowledge the concern that industrial funding may bias researchers and lead to bias in published data, which in turn may lead to erroneous recommendations for clinical practice. But we should be more concerned about the conflict of interest that is created when clinician-researchers are given incentives to sell their patients to industry. . . . Patients come to academic medical centers trusting that their physicians are focused on their interests; they do not come to help us promote industry's research agenda. . . . The interjection of industry into the doctor-patient relationship is disturbing; worse, patients often are not aware of its presence."[7]

THE CONCERN, of course, is that drug-company influences will reduce the accuracy and reliability of drug research, thereby reducing drug safety. This concern is realistic: It has been shown that studies funded by drug companies provide favorable results for the companies' products significantly more often than studies conducted independently.[8,9] For example, an analysis of seventy studies on the safety of calcium-channel blockers (antagonists) concluded that "authors who supported the use of calcium-channel antagonists were significantly more likely than neutral or critical authors to have financial relationships with manufacturers of calcium-channel antagonists." Ninety-six percent of authors with drug-company ties viewed the safety profile of these drugs favorably, while only 37 percent without such ties viewed their safety favorably. The report added: "Our results demonstrate a strong association between authors' published positions . . . and their financial relationships with pharmaceutical manufacturers. The medical profession needs to develop a more effective policy on conflict of interest."[10]

Drug-company-supported studies on cancer drugs reported unfavorable conclusions only 5 percent of the time; yet, when independent studies were conducted, unfavorable conclusions were reported 38 percent of the time.[11] The accurate reporting of side effects and other problems with cancer drugs is essential for the comfort and safety of chemotherapy patients. Slanted data jeopardizes patients' welfare and comfort.

In a 2000 article in *Medical Hypotheses,* researchers condemned the influence of drug companies on multiple sclerosis research. "It has to be emphasized that the degree to which the biomedical industry can influence and control academic research and publications, as well as clinical practice . . . has now become a severe problem. . . . A new set of ethical requirements, limiting the ability of the biomedical industry to influence, interfere with, and/or control academic research and publications should be agreed upon."[12]

In an interview with the Associated Press, Dr. Thomas Bodenheimer, a clinical professor in the department of family and community medicine at the University of California, San Francisco, listed other serious biases in drug-company-sponsored studies such as selectively reporting only the good results in a drug trial, making claims not justified by the evidence, and "outright fraud with fabrication of evidence." He added, "Investigators who allow bias or error to affect their work are practicing scientific misconduct."[13]

Dr. Ian Chalmers, a respected expert on medical ethics, raised similar concerns ten years earlier: "Failure to publish an adequate account of a well-designed clinical trial is a form of scientific misconduct that can lead those caring for patients to make inappropriate treatment decisions."[14]

DRUG COMPANIES CAN exert the most influence on studies conducted within the companies themselves or when contracting with a new industry of commercial research organizations established specifically to cater to drug-company interests. These for-profit commercial organizations allow drug companies considerable leeway in writing their own study designs and in performing their own analyses of the results. Dr. Bodenheimer addressed these issues in an article titled "Uneasy Alliance: Clinical Investigators and the Pharmaceutical Industry" in *The New England Journal of Medicine* in May 2000. Reporting findings from interviews of thirty-nine experts, Bodenheimer presented a disturbing list of worrisome trends. Several experts stated that the drug companies' control over research data allows them to "provide the spin on the data that favors them." Bodenheimer reported that some commercial research organizations "have been criticized for producing data of poor quality and inadequately training investigators." Other experts viewed commercial research organizations as "the handmaidens of pharmaceutical companies, concerned with the approval and marketing of drugs rather than with true science."[15]

Because of the many advantages that commercial research organizations provide the pharmaceutical industry, drug companies have funneled huge sums of money to them while drastically cutting monies to academic medical institutions, further squeezing medical centers into compliance with drug-company goals.

THERE ARE MANY SUBTLE ways by which drug companies can slant study designs in their favor. One method is for a drug company to compare its new drug at a potent dose against a competitor's drug at a less effective dose.[16] Drs. Paula Rochon and Jeffrey Gurwitz found this was the case in 48 percent of the studies they reviewed for a new anti-inflammatory drug.[17] Such methods make the new drug appear superior, although it really isn't. The drug company can then advertise the drug's "superiority."

Drug companies can define effectiveness in a number of ways, allowing them to select the best results for influencing doctors while discarding less impressive results.[18] Drug companies can choose between study designs, avoiding more accurate designs if the results may reveal limited effectiveness of drugs or unsatisfactory numbers of side effects. This may explain why "51% of approved drugs have serious adverse effects not detected prior to approval," according to Dr. Thomas Moore of George Washington University. "The discovery of new dangers of drugs after marketing is common."[19]

To ensure favorable profiles for their drugs, drug companies have many ways of dealing with unfavorable findings. According to Dr. Chalmers, substantial numbers of studies are never published at all.[20] Or drug companies can create delays in analyzing the data for publication—delays so lengthy that it renders the results irrelevant or impossible to publish.[21] During these delays, some companies have conducted secret studies that provide better results; these are rushed into publication in order to invalidate the original unfavorable findings.[22]

Researchers who push to publish unfavorable findings in order to warn the public have been threatened with loss of funding, lawsuits, or blacklisting from future drug-company studies. "When Dr. Nancy Oliveri at the University of Toronto wanted to warn patients about toxic side effects of a drug she was testing, the company supporting her research tried to quash her findings, citing a nondisclosure agreement," according to a 1999 article in the *Los Angeles Times*.[23] Oliveri alerted her patients anyway. The drug company suspended the clinical trial and canceled her research contract. Undeterred, she published her concerns. The hospital in which she worked dismissed her, according to the *Times*. This triggered an international protest. Supported by faculty groups and health-care experts, Oliveri won reinstatement. But she had learned the lesson: "I will never ever again accept drug company money that is not clearly and completely free of any secrecy clauses whatsoever."[24]

The Oliveri incident wasn't unique. University of California, San Francisco, researcher Dr. Betty Dong found evidence that disputed the effectiveness of a top-selling thyroid medication purchased by six million Americans each year.[25,26] This was vital information, but Dong had signed a nondisclosure agreement as part of her funding. "It made me nervous," she said, "but evidently a lot of people sign these clauses." The drug company was able to block publication of her findings for seven years.[27]

When Dr. James Khan's study concluded that a new vaccine didn't help AIDS patients, the corporation funding his work tried to block publication of the unfavorable results. When Dr. Khan published the study, the corporation sued Dr. Kahn and the University of California at San Francisco. "In light of such intimidation," Dr. Bodenheimer commented, "few researchers will have the courage to stand up to the companies that fund them."[28]

One experienced researcher told Dr. Bodenheimer, "When results favor the drug company, everything is great. But when results are disappointing, there is commonly an effort to spin, downplay, or change findings."[29] Dr. Curt Furberg, Professor of Public Health Sciences at Wake Forest University School of Medicine, added, "Companies can play hardball, and many investigators can't play hardball back. You send the paper to the company for comments, and that's the danger. Can you handle the changes the company wants? Will you give in a little, a little more, then capitulate? It's tricky for those who need money for more studies."[30]

And more than ever, research physicians depend on drug-company money, for while drug-company profits have skyrocketed, so has their leverage on financially beleaguered medical institutions and their faculty members. Yet, these financial ties are often hidden even from patients induced to volunteer in studies of new drugs. In a March 2001 article in the *Seattle Times* titled "The Ethical Dilemmas of Drugs, Money, Medicine," Dr. Bodenheimer and Ronald Collins, of the Center for Science in the Public Interest, wrote, "Researchers do not regularly divulge their financial ties to drug companies when asking patients to enroll in drug trials. Financial conflict of interest in clinical drug trials is a significant problem in the United States. It affects millions of people—those who are subjects in drug trials and those who use the drugs once they enter the market. . . . Predictably, company-funded research tends to favor company products."[31]

DR. RAYMOND WOOSLEY, the chairman of the Department of Pharmacology at Georgetown University, has a solution. For years he has sought funding for an independent national research center where unbiased, in-depth studies of drugs' effectiveness and safety can be conducted. A center is needed because many important drug studies are never conducted. The drug companies, Woosley told *The Wall Street Journal* in December 1999, "fund research that has the potential to establish or improve a drug's place in the market."[32] Other experts agree, including Harvard's Jerry Avorn: "Industry-sponsored research does not necessarily address many important clinical and policy problems."[33] "Companies put huge amounts of money in trials directed toward their interests," Dr. Stuart Pocock told *The New York Times* in December 2000. "And their interests are, in general, in danger of being in conflict with what are society's interests."[34]

The same situation exists in Europe. In a 2000 *British Medical Journal* article titled "The risk of bias from omitted research: evidence must be independently sought and free of economic interests," Italian researchers Silvio Garattini and Alessandro Liberati wrote, "It is unfortunate that industrialized countries . . . have delegated the control of drug trials to pharmaceutical companies. We are not suggesting that the industry is wicked, and we acknowledge its role in providing essential drugs. . . . Nevertheless, delegating this responsibility places clear limitations on research, and they seem to be growing."[35]

But, as *The Wall Street Journal* reported, "not everyone is thrilled" with Dr. Woosley's proposal for an independent national drug-research center, "and even some proponents are only nervously optimistic. . . . One reason for such skittishness is that the push into so-called effectiveness studies could run counter to the interests of big drug companies. . . ." Physicians depending on drug-company funding were wary because "they may inadvertently antagonize the drug companies—a potentially risky proposition."[36]

Woosley confessed nervousness too. "I'll be honest. I don't want to offend the drug industry. I think we can do a lot of work to help people use drugs more effectively without directly attacking somebody's market. . . . If you start ranking drugs as one better than the other, then you start making people mad and your funding is cut. But I don't want to roll over, either."[37]

But ranking drugs according to their effectiveness and safety is exactly what is needed. Such head-to-head comparisons are done every day with other products. *Consumer Reports,* which publishes comparative analyses of automobiles and home products every month, serves a vital role and, therefore, is one of the most successful magazines ever. Yet, with medications, no one dares challenge the drug companies. If a researcher as established as Dr. Woosley has to tread cautiously when discussing the vital need for independent studies, it speaks volumes about how beholden and dependent the rest of the research community is on the drug industry.

In 1999, after years of resistance, Dr. Woosley obtained government funding for his research center: a mere $2.5 million of his request for $75 million—and a pittance compared to the billions controlled by the drug companies.[38]

Failing to Complete Research Required by the FDA

Sometimes, when the research isn't sufficient, the FDA approves new drugs with the understanding that the drug companies will conduct further studies. However, according to Ralph Nader's watchdog agency, Public Citizen, "Data obtained from the Food and Drug Administration through a Freedom of Information Act (FOIA) request shows that drug companies are failing to fulfill their post-marketing research (Phase 4) commitments." In fact, of the 88 drugs approved between 1990 and 1994 with at least one commitment for further study, only 11 of these drugs (13 percent) were listed as completed by the FDA by late 1999. Of the 107 drugs approved since January 1995, not one had completed its promised post-approval study as of June 2000. Public Citizen concluded: "This result suggests grossly inadequate compliance by drug companies in meeting their Phase 4 [post-approval] study commitments."[39]

Public Citizen also surveyed physicians working for the FDA. Regarding the drug companies' record with follow-up studies, one FDA officer stated: "We don't trust that the companies will carry out Phase 4 studies with due diligence." Another wrote: "My office director told me that he was going to overrule me because the sponsor [a drug company] would just go over our heads to Capitol Hill. He felt it was best to approve the drug for an indication not studied and have the sponsors do a Phase 4 post-marketing trial in support of the indication. I reminded him that this sponsor had failed to honor other Phase 4 studies. He went ahead and approved the drug."[40]

Unfortunately, the FDA's powers to enforce many of its requirements are limited, thanks to constraints by Congress. Perhaps not coincidentally, drug companies contribute heavily for lobbying and political contributions. The drug industry employs hundreds of lobbyists and gives millions to the political parties and to congressional and presidential candidates.[41] Critics of the drug companies in Congress are few. As former Senator Slade Gorton told *The New York Times* in October 2000, "They are extremely reluctant to step out as I have, because they don't want to be trashed."[42]

THE RESULT OF all of these problems is unsafe drugs, unnecessary drugs, unreliable information—and improper dosages. In 2001, Dr. Peck, a former FDA section director and now the director of the

Center of Drug Development Science at Georgetown University, and Dr. James Cross of the FDA reported that 22 percent of all drugs approved between 1980 and 1999 required changes in their dosage guidelines. Most of these changes were reductions in dosages prompted by reports to the FDA of side effects in patients.[43] Thus, for these drugs, proper dosages were determined not during early research, as they should have been, but only after the overmedication of unsuspecting patients. Furthermore, belatedly reducing the recommended dosages of drugs years after they were approved usually does little to change doctors from prescribing higher dosages, because once doctors have learned the original recommended doses, they usually don't read the package inserts or PDR again, so they keep prescribing the higher doses, and patients continue to be overmedicated.

Moreover, the drugs reported by Dr. Peck and Dr. Cross represent only the tip of the iceberg, for they do not include many of the medications discussed in this book. Effective, safer, lower doses of top-selling drugs such as Prozac, Voltaren, Celebrex, Lipitor, many antihypertensive drugs, etc., have yet to be widely recognized, and important low-dose information has yet to be provided in drug-company product information or many drug references.

Moreover, the problem is getting worse. A drug approved between 1995 and 1999 was twice as likely to have its dosage changed as a drug approved between 1980 and 1984. Dr. Peck stated, "Consumers should understand that drug companies and the FDA do the best they can to get the dose right at the beginning of marketing. However, because of the need to develop drugs fast so they can get the drugs out to those who need them, there is the expectation that the dosage information will be improved over time. So consumers should also be aware that the doses might be either too high or too low for any individual." In other words, you can't rely on the dosages that the drug companies recommend to doctors and that doctors prescribe to you. This is an absurd, unacceptable situation. As Dr. Peck stated in 1997 in the *Food Drug Law Journal:* "Post-marketing dosage changes reflect a flaw in the traditional paradigm for drug development."[44] This "flaw" has yet to be corrected—indeed, it is getting worse—and the result is the continuing side-effect epidemic.

Deceptive Publishing Strategies

Drug companies exert considerable efforts in pushing their products to physicians, the media, and the public. Their tactics are many.

In a 1999 *JAMA* article titled "Fair Conduct and Fair Reporting of Clinical Trials," Dr. Drummond Rennie, a deputy editor at *JAMA,* described how companies magnify unimpressive results in drug studies by analyzing the results in multiple ways, then publishing these results under the names of different authors in different medical journals.[45] This provides the impression that the favorable data on a drug are substantial. A 1996 article in *Lancet* noted: "Multiple renditions of the same information is self-serving, wasteful . . . and can be profoundly misleading; it brings into question the integrity of medical research."[46] Dr. Rennie added, "The evidence shows that covert reporting of the same data in clinical trials artificially skews the balance of opinion in favor of a new drug. Why is this happening? Reviewing these case studies, it is hard not to suspect that this practice, which serves commercial interests so well, is deliberate and, because it confuses and biases information important to the care of patients, it has to stop."[47] So far, it hasn't.

Other tactics include hiring professional writers to prepare articles to drug-company specifications and advantage. In the past, medical researchers analyzed their findings objectively and published the results themselves. Today, drug companies hire professional writers— ghostwriters—who are neither physicians nor have been involved in the studies. Dr. Bodenheimer explained, "Ghostwriters typically receive a packet of materials from which they write the article. They may be instructed to insert a key paragraph favorable to the company's product."[48]

In a 1999 article in *Lancet,* medical writer Ronni Sandroff described how a drug company paid her for two articles about cancer treatments. These articles would not be published under her name but under the names of prestigious doctors. "I was told exactly what the drug company expected and given explicit instructions about what to play up and what to play down. . . ." Writer Marilynn Larkin recounted, "I recently had my first and last experience as a 'ghostwriter' . . . for a supplement to appear under the names of respected authors. I was given an outline, references, and a list of drug-company approved phrases. I was asked to sign an agreement stating that I would not disclose anything about the project. I was pressured to rework my drafts to position the product more favorably, and was shown another company-produced review as an example—it read like bad promotional writing."[49]

Unfortunately, it is not uncommon for respected physicians to accept drug-company money to lend their names to research they had nothing to do with. "The practice is well-known, scandalous, and outrageous," Dr. Drummond Rennie wrote in *Lancet.* "It is a perfect illustration of deceptive authorship practices for commercial reasons."[50]

Harvard School of Public Health physician Troyen Brennan provided an in-depth description in *The New England Journal of Medicine* of how respected physicians are recruited as figurehead authors—ghost authors—for drug-company-sponsored articles.[51] One day, Brennan received a call from a public relations firm offering him $2,500, provided by a drug company, to "author" an article. Brennan would merely have to discuss the subject with a ghostwriter and then review the ghostwritten draft. Brennan played along and was sent a promotional packet describing how drug-company-funded public relations firms keep drug sales brisk via intensive advertising, special symposiums led by paid experts, and "management of the press." In addition, the drug companies underwrote articles for medical journals, but without disclosing the authors' actual source of funding.

Dr. Brennan's experience wasn't an exception. In an article in *JAMA*, several *JAMA* editors wrote: "Approximately 1 in 4 articles [in six top medical journals] demonstrated misapplication of authorship criteria and inappropriate assignment of authorship." The authors termed these practices "incompatible with the principles, duties, and ethical responsibilities involved in scientific publication."[52] An article published in April 2001 revealed that of more than 61,000 articles published in 181 academic journals in 1997, only one half of 1 percent detailed the authors' personal financial interests, although it is believed that up to 50 percent of academic physicians consult with the drug industry. Scientists who do not report conflicts of interest usually "believe that they are people of integrity, and they feel they can separate their work from their financial interests," Dr. David Blumenthal, director of the Institute for Health Policy at Massachusetts General Hospital, told *The New York Times*. However, studies have shown that physicians with financial ties to the drug industry tend to write more favorably about the industry's products.[53]

Brennan warned: "The problem of conflicts of interest will probably only grow worse in the years ahead." He called for stronger rules that would require all journal article authors to reveal their sources of funding. He also discussed the appropriateness of banning articles by authors with severe conflicts of interest, but he concluded this was impractical because "too many academic physicians depend on funding from for-profit firms, especially drug companies."[54]

If the influence of the drug companies on medical research is so extensive that the medical profession cannot even attempt to ensure the objectivity of its own experts, we are indeed scraping bottom. This isn't merely a problem of ivory tower academics—it affects everyday patients. "Real patients suffer real harm from biased studies that offer false or incomplete information, including information about a doctor's financial ties to a pharmaceutical company," wrote Dr. Bodenheimer and Ronald Collins, of the Center for Science in the Public Interest, in March 2001.[55]

PERHAPS ALL INDUSTRIES manipulate facts to their advantage, but these drug-company practices ultimately harm people. For instance, a May 1999 front-page headline read: "Maker of Fen-Phen Paid for Articles: Lawsuit Says Wyeth Hid Dangers Linked to Weight-Loss Drugs." The Associated Press article reported:

A company that manufactured part of the diet drug combination fen-phen hired ghostwriters for articles promoting obesity treatment and then used prominent researchers to publish the works under their names, according to lawsuit evidence cited in a newspaper report yesterday. The legal action contends that Wyeth-Ayerst Laboratories, which made the 'fen' half of the drug combination, hid health risks associated with the drugs. The company allegedly tried to play down or remove descriptions of side effects from articles, *The Dallas Morning News* reported.[56]

A spokesman for Wyeth described this as "a common practice in the industry. . . . The companies have some input . . . but the proposed author has the last say." However, the University of Pennsylvania's Dr. Albert Stunkard, one of the researchers involved, said he hadn't known that Wyeth financed or edited his article. Had he known, he would not have participated. "It's really deceptive," he said.[57]

Asked about these practices, Dr. Robert Terney Jr., chairman of the AMA's council on ethical and judicial affairs, stated, "What they're doing here is clearly an advertisement, but it's couched as a scientifically valid paper."[58]

Furthermore, according to the lawsuit, Wyeth hired a company to write as many as ten articles on the diet drugs. The company then planned to submit some of the papers to medical journals owned by Wyeth's parent company, Reed Elsevier plc, the Associated Press reported.[59]

Gifts and Other Perquisites for Physicians

Drug companies have always tried to influence doctors to select their products, but today their influence is greater than ever. Drug companies spend an average of $13,000 for each doctor—totaling $8 billion annually—to gain access and influence with physicians through sales personnel and advertising.[60]

Drug companies maintain a force of 70,000 sales representatives who visit doctors' offices to make pitches for their products.[61] In the hospitals, drug sales representatives target new doctors, particularly interns and residents. Knowing that these overworked people are frequently underpaid and usually in debt, they offer dinners, gifts, difficult-to-obtain tickets, and other inducements as ways of forging relationships and exerting influence that will continue when these physicians enter practice. The payoff for the drug companies? As a medical resident told ABC News: "We have no choice but to listen to their biased information."[62]

They do have a choice, of course, but accepting these drug-company overtures has become such an ingrained part of the medical system, doing so seems normal and refusing appears peevish.

IF BIASED SALES pitches to interns and residents were the only attempts by drug companies to influence physicians, it might not be so bad. But when drug companies spend money on doctors—for gifts, meetings, sporting events, travel, lodging, and educational symposia—more prescriptions are written for the companies' drugs.[63] A 2000 study in *JAMA* found:

> Attending sponsored continuing medical education events and accepting funding for travel or lodging for educational symposia were associated with increased prescription rates of the sponsor's medication. Attending presentations given by pharmaceutical representative speakers was also associated with nonrational prescribing. Conclusion: The present extent of physician-industry interactions appears to affect prescribing and professional behavior and should be further addressed at the level of policy and education.[64]

By "nonrational prescribing" the article meant that doctors were prescribing drugs that were more expensive, less effective, or both. In some cases, doctors were more likely—sometimes twenty times more likely—to request the addition of drug-company–sponsored drugs to hospital formularies, even though most of the requested drugs "presented little or no therapeutic advantage."[65]

When meetings are sponsored by drug companies, the content may be biased toward the sponsors' products.[66] Dr. J. W. Norton, of the University of Mississippi Medical Center, provided a glimpse of how drug companies select physicians willing to present the companies' points of view. In a letter to *The New England Journal of Medicine,* Dr. Norton described being invited by a drug company to lecture. "In my attempts to present balanced information, I deluded myself into thinking I was educating physicians, not being swayed by the sponsors." Dr. Norton made the mistake of writing that a drug by the sponsor caused more side effects than a competitor's drug. "My invitations to speak suddenly dropped from 4–6 times per month to essentially none." Worried about the loss of income, "I found myself seeking out representatives of the company to let them know I was still 'on the team.' I began to worry that I was not prescribing enough of their medication. I was amazed at how I had become seduced by pressure to be kind to the sponsor's product. This experience has opened my eyes, and I will proceed with caution—that is, if I am ever invited to be a speaker again."[67]

Although some doctors recognize the dangers of receiving drug company "gifts," some don't. They are offended when it is implied that any influence could alter their commitment to scientific principles and to prescribing only the best medication for every patient. But studies in physicians' behavior prove them wrong. Dr. A. Wazana of McGill University stated in *JAMA,* "Although most physicians report paying little attention to drug advertising and pharmaceutical representatives, their [actions] revealed their receptivity to commercial sources."[68] Ethical guidelines suggest that all gifts from drug companies to doctors should serve an educational purpose and not be of "substantial" value ($100), but these guidelines are voluntary, and the AMA now concedes that doctors are increasingly ignoring them.[69]

Dr. Robert Tenery, American Medical Association Counsel on Ethical and Judicial Affairs, described the intensification of drug company influence:

Although the business interests of the pharmaceutical industry have always potentially conflicted with the best interests of patients, it is only since the 1980s that these conflicts threatened to adversely affect patient care. In addition to promoting name recognition and access to prescribers, the pharmaceutical industry has created incentives that, in themselves, alter prescribing habits." These practices are "so effective that many physicians are not even aware of the influence of these techniques on their own behavior.[70]

These abuses continue because doctors have never adopted the strict rules of accountability established by other professions. For example, the media operates within clearly defined rules regarding conflicts of interest. One senior editor of a major publication told me, "I am shocked at the conflicts of interest that are allowed in the medical profession. If I had any type of financial arrangement with a company or simply owned stock in it, I would not be allowed to involve myself in any article that discussed the company. Company policies and our own ethics don't allow it. I could be demoted or fired."

A financial adviser told me, "The Securities and Exchange Commission has very tight rules about financial or consulting arrangements. If I have any links whatsoever to a company, I cannot write an article or analysis of the company's standing. If I did, I could lose my license."

But no doctor loses his license, or even faces a fine or censure, for similar conflicts of interest in today's medical-pharmaceutical complex. Quite the contrary: For many doctors today, making as many financial arrangements with drug companies as possible is the road to success.

Controlling Information to Physicians and Consumers

The drug companies also influence physicians by being their main source of drug information, and one of the drug companies' foremost instruments is the *Physicians' Desk Reference.* All of the information in the *PDR* is written by the drug companies, and it is with drug industry support that this expensive volume is delivered free each year to every practicing doctor in the United States. First published in 1947 as a promotional device, today more than 90 percent of physicians consult the *PDR* when making prescribing decisions.[71,72] Eighty-two percent of doctors regard the *PDR* as their single most useful drug reference. Overall, doctors refer to the *PDR* 265,000,000 times a year.

The *PDR* does contain some very good information, but the book isn't a true drug reference. A true reference contains information from independent sources as well as from drug manufacturers. It contains updated information from medical journals and symposia, not just drug company–designed studies. A true drug reference compares the different medications for common disorders, and it makes recommendations for selecting the best drugs and dosages for each clinical problem.

The *PDR* does none of these. That's because the *PDR* is almost entirely composed of package inserts, which mainly reflect the early research on new drugs that the drug companies conducted in order to obtain FDA approval. As I have pointed out in articles in the *Archives of Internal Medicine*,[73–75] *Postgraduate Medicine*,[76] and *Geriatrics*,[77] the *PDR* contains little Phase 4 information—the more comprehensive, more recent, more accurate, largely independently accrued postapproval information from the usage of medications in millions of people over many years.

This is why the *PDR* does not mention many standard uses of drugs such as Prozac for panic disorder or social phobia, or Celebrex for tendinitis or menstrual pain. This is why the *PDR* does not reflect many new side effects or the lower, safer, initial doses of scores of drugs that are discovered after FDA approval. This is why for decades the *PDR* has recommended unnecessarily high doses of Premarin and HCTZ, and why the *PDR* still says little or nothing about low-dose Prilosec, Voltaren, Lipitor, Celebrex, and many other top-selling drugs. This is why more than a decade of new *PDR*'s have kept reporting the same old, understated statistics for sexual dysfunctions with Prozac. In fact, there is no formal mechanism by which drug companies are required to regularly update the information in the *PDR*. Instead, major changes in the *PDR* require FDA approval—a sometimes lengthy step that presents a further barrier to keeping the *PDR* current.

Yet, the *PDR* is almost ubiquitous in physicians' offices as well as on hospital floors, where it is frequently used by residents and interns. Nurses and other health professionals also rely on the *PDR*. The *PDR*'s high profile is the result of intense marketing that sends the volume free to 500,000 physicians, hospitals, and libraries a year. The *PDR* also influences consumers who purchase more than half a million copies from bookstores annually. It also influences people who buy other consumer references, because a large amount of the information in these references is derived from the *PDR*. However, many people— health professionals and consumers alike—are unaware of the deficiencies of the *PDR* or that its information and recommendations may lead to suboptimal care. They have no idea that the *PDR* information does not reflect a great deal of important, more current information published in medical journals.

An example of the *PDR*'s limitations was revealed in a 1997 article titled "Incorrect Overdose Management Advice in the *Physicians' Desk Reference*" in the *Annals of Emergency Medicine*.[78] In the article, researchers reported the results of an analysis of the *PDR*'s overdose guidelines for twenty medications commonly used for suicide attempts. Of all the data the *PDR* contains, it would be expected that this vital information would be kept the most current. The authors found quite the opposite.

We found serious discrepancies in overdose treatment advice in the PDR compared with a consensus of current toxicology references. Altogether, four of every five PDR entries [i.e., 16 of the 20 drugs studied] were deficient, and almost half advised ineffective or frankly contraindicated therapies. Despite FDA approval, the use of PDR overdose advice in a serious poisoning case could result in unnecessary morbidity or mortality.[79]

Because the *PDR* is published in a new edition each year, people assume that it reflects the current state of medical knowledge about the *PDR*'s hundreds of listed drugs. Clearly, this is not necessarily the case.

The issue here is not that the *PDR* contains drug company information or that it is disseminated to doctors with pharmaceutical industry support. The issue is that by aggressively marketing the *PDR*, the drug companies have made this book—a book that has never risen to the standards of a true drug reference—the dominant written source of drug information for physicians. Moreover, because of the annual, free dissemination of the *PDR* to physicians, true drug references have not been able to compete with the *PDR*. The *AMA Drug Evaluations,* perhaps the foremost independent drug reference, sold only 16,000 volumes in 1994 at more than $100 apiece.[80] In 1996, the *AMA Drug Evaluations* ceased publication. The *American Hospital Formulary Service Drug Information* is an excellent, up-to-date, comprehensive reference, but it is sold primarily to pharmacies. Relatively few physicians purchase it. Many pharmacists have told me that they rarely use the *PDR* and greatly prefer *Drug Facts and Comparisons,* but I've never met a physician who uses it.

In order to provide optimal treatment to patients, physicians must have a readily available source of current, comprehensive, accurate information. The dominance of the *PDR* has had the opposite effect— it has rendered physicians reliant on its limited information. If new dosing methods or new treatment possibilities are not mentioned in the *PDR,* many physicians will not know about them. Medical journals offer this information, but there are hundreds of journals and most physicians read just a few. Without a recognized, reliable source of complete, independent, up-to-date information, there is nowhere for physicians or other healthcare professionals to turn. Then, physicians' knowledge and methods do not keep pace. Thus, it is not surprising that a March 2001 report by the Institute of Medicine showed it can take seventeen years for important medical discoveries to become accepted and extensively used by office physicians.[81]

This will not change until physicians and patients have ready access to a complete, comprehensive, current drug reference. Perhaps, as I have suggested in several of my journal articles, the *PDR* can be improved to fulfill this role. Perhaps the drug industry, government, and medical experts can develop mechanisms by which this can be achieved. Otherwise, the free dissemination of the *PDR* to physicians should be discouraged, and physicians and consumers should turn to a more complete source of medication information.

THE *PDR,* free meetings and gifts, and direct contact by drug-company representatives constitute three major ways that drug companies influence physicians' choices of medications. A fourth way is advertising. Most of this advertising is done in medical journals, which also serve as an important source of information for physicians.

A cursory look at almost any medical journal will reveal dozens of advertisements by the drug companies. Glossy ads promote the efficacy or ease of usage of drugs. Some ads boast that physicians don't have to bother reducing the drugs' dosages for older people, not even for those with other disorders or taking other medication. The content of these ads is based on the information in package inserts, with the same limitations or omissions of important side effects and/or lower, safer doses.

Remarkably, despite heavy reliance on revenues from drug-company advertising, most medical journals have remained relatively independent in their choices of articles to publish. In fact, some journals such as *JAMA,* the *British Medical Journal,* the *Archives of Internal Medicine,* and *The New England Journal of Medicine* have published many articles focusing on the growing influence of the pharmaceutical industry on every aspect of the medical profession.

But this, too, may be changing. At *The New England Journal of Medicine,* Dr. Marcia Angell is no longer editor in chief. Dr. Angell was serving as the temporary editor in chief after the former editor in chief, Dr. Jeffrey Kassirer, was fired because, according to the *Los Angeles Times,* "he balked at plans to leverage the journal's name and logo to promote other products."[82] Angell applied for the permanent position, but the board of directors chose Dr. Jeffrey Drazen, a respected researcher with long-established ties with the drug industry.[83,84]

The decision wasn't entirely surprising. According to a May 2000 article in *The New York Times,* "In recent years, the journal has become a huge source of revenue for the [Massachusetts] medical society, largely through increased drug company advertising."[85] And the society no longer publishes its profits, which have risen tremendously.

Because of concerns about conflicts of interest, Dr. Drazen agreed to recuse himself from some editorial activities, but he still is empowered to make the final decisions about a wide range of issues and to hire and dismiss other editors and staff. In other words, while Dr. Drazen will likely make a good-faith effort to be objective, his long experience and apparent comfort with the pharmaceutical industry may influence his staffing and publishing decisions, thereby altering the tone of the famous journal.

With so many physicians having financial connections with the pharmaceutical industry, is it inevitable that top positions at major journals will be increasingly filled with drug-industry–sympathetic people? Already, because of ghostwriters and ghost authors and undisclosed conflicts of interest, medical journals are having difficulty ensuring the integrity of their articles. A front-page story in the February 25, 2000, *Los Angeles Times* described how *The New England Journal of Medicine*, "the world's most influential medical journal, has admitted to an extraordinary betrayal of its own ethics, saying that nearly half of the drug reviews published since 1997 were written by researchers with undisclosed financial support from companies marketing the drugs. . . . The ethical breach also shows the deep inroads that commercial sponsorship has made into academic research and publishing."[86]

"It's symptomatic of where the money comes from nowadays to do research in medicine," Mildred Cho, a research scholar at the Stanford University Center for Biomedical Ethics, told the newspaper.[87]

THE DANGERS of all of these drug-company influences is revealed when physicians prescribe new drugs with extra risks and no advantages over established medications to millions of people. Duract, a new anti-inflammatory drug introduced in 1997, is one of many examples.

Duract was similar to aspirin and a dozen other, more proven anti-inflammatory drugs that were already available. However, Duract did differ from the others in one important respect—the severity of its effects on the liver.[88,89] According to the *Boston Globe:*

Early testing revealed that Duract could damage the liver, and this did not escape the attention of veteran FDA medical reviewer Richard Widmark. He noted that some other drugs in this family had also shown liver toxicity, but concluded Duract was the worst he had seen.[90]

After its release, Duract was promptly linked with liver toxicities and deaths. With safer alternative drugs available, there was no basis for doctors to prescribe Duract, yet doctors were persuaded to prescribe the drug million of times. The author of the *Boston Globe* article, Dr. Thomas Moore, of the Center for Health Policy Research at George Washington University Medical Center, wrote: "So effective is the industry at marketing, and so uncritical are prescribing physicians, that more than 2.5 million prescriptions of Duract were written in the 10 months before Duract was withdrawn because of the expected, predictable, and entirely preventable liver deaths."[91]

In a powerful editorial in *JAMA* discussing Duract and other withdrawn drugs, Dr. Alastair Wood, assistant vice chancellor for research at the Vanderbilt University Medical Center, declared that physicians "should resist marketing pressures to prescribe new and potentially more toxic drugs in preference to prescribing well-established safer drugs."[92] He added, "Manufacturers should behave responsibly in the promotion of new drugs for which toxicity is, by definition, currently unknown."

BUT CONCERNED PHYSICIANS have been saying these things for decades. I remember when Valium was introduced in the 1960's as a "nonaddictive" alternative to the barbiturates. But, of course, Valium proved to cause severe dependency reactions when prescribed at unnecessarily high doses. This problem harmed a lot of people, but it didn't harm Roche Labs, which profited immensely from Valium's worldwide top-selling status for over a decade.

When Valium's dangers were finally revealed and the public became wary of the drug, I watched closely, amazed and appalled, as Xanax burst onto the scene as the new, "safer" Valium. Obviously intending to fill the huge Valium market, Upjohn launched a torrent of advertising that emphasized Xanax's superiority over Valium. Although

Xanax belonged to the same chemical family as Valium, doctors quickly made Xanax a best-seller. But to any doctor who remembered his basic science, it was apparent that Xanax might be less safe than Valium, because fast-acting and fast-departing drugs like Xanax are usually more prone to dependency and withdrawal reactions than slowly metabolized drugs like Valium.

In fact, I saw far more dependency, more quickly, and of greater severity with Xanax than ever with Valium. Although I prescribed Xanax very carefully—it does have benefits when used correctly—even at the very lowest manufacturer-recommended doses, some of my patients developed dependency and withdrawal problems. Patients of other doctors began showing up at my office on unbelievably high, addicting doses of Xanax, suffering withdrawal reactions even though they were still taking the drug. This horror show motivated me to write my first articles and letters challenging our methods of producing and prescribing medications. This was in 1987.

Today, experts continue writing about withdrawal problems with Xanax, as reflected in a March 2001 article in Primary Psychiatry by its editor, Dr. Norman Sussman: "Short half-life benzodiazepines, such as alprazolam [Xanax] and lorazepam [Ativan], are associated with more frequent and severe withdrawal symptoms, even between doses."[93] The 2000 PDR now offers more than 140 lines of information in its "Warnings" section about withdrawal with Xanax, including this: "Certain adverse clinical events, some life-threatening, are a direct consequence of physical dependence on Xanax. Even after relatively short-term use at the dose recommended for the treatment of transient anxiety and anxiety disorder (i.e., 0.75 to 4.0 mg per day), there is some risk of dependence."[94] At the same time, the Xanax dosage guidelines continue to recommend doses that I consider too high—and Xanax and its generic, alprazolam, continue to sell briskly.

Zyban is heavily advertised as a solution for people wanting to stop smoking. But Zyban isn't new at all: It is Wellbutrin, an antidepressant that's been around for a decade. Does Zyban work? In a few people. The studies that accompanied Zyban's highly orchestrated, well-advertised introduction showed that twenty-six weeks after use of Zyban, only 19 percent of patients remained off cigarettes. The placebo treatment used in the study worked for 11 percent—in other words, Zyban produced a mere 8-percent improvement over placebo.[95] Curious about this unimpressive result, in 1998 I obtained a summary of Zyban's studies from GlaxoWellcome.[96] In one study, only 13 percent of Zyban users had remained off cigarettes continuously for 52 weeks, just 3 percent better than placebo. In another, 23 percent had remained off cigarettes continuously for 52 weeks, 15 percent better than placebo.

Do these numbers make Zyban worthy of such prodigious advertising? Maybe not, especially when the February 2001 edition of the *British Medical Journal* reported that Zyban had been linked to 3,457 reports of adverse reactions including several cases of seizures and eighteen deaths in Britain.[97] Whether or not Zyban was the cause wasn't known, but GlaxoWellcome states that the incidence of seizures is 1 in 1,000 patients taking the standard dosage of Zyban.[98]

Xenical, the new diet drug, is advertised frequently too. The drug-company dosage: 120 mg three times a day—for everyone. It doesn't matter if you are 18 or 81 years old, or if you weigh 115 pounds or 350 pounds—you receive the same dose. The manufacturer describes most of Xenical's side effects as minor. Not everyone would agree. In the manufacturer's own studies, patients taking Xenical reported: greasy flatulence in 24 percent of patients, oily spotting of underwear in 27 percent, urgent need for a bowel movement in 22 percent, fatty or oily stools in 20 percent, increased defecation in 11 percent, and fecal incontinence in 8 percent. Xenical can cause other problems, but just counting these adds up to a total of 112 potential side effects per 100 people.[99]

If you are still interested in taking Xenical—which does work for some people—you may think it wise to try a lower dose first, just to test your sensitivity and avoid an embarrassing experience. But Roche Labs doesn't agree, for it recommends Xenical at a one-size-fits-all dosage of 120 mg three times a day with each meal and produces Xenical in only a one-size 120-mg capsule—despite studies showing that a 50 percent lower Xenical dosage, 60 mg three times a day, was significantly effective.[100–102]

Physicians certainly deserve their share of responsibility for these problems in drug use and the resultant side-effect epidemic. But the problems begin with the drug companies' research methods; with their attempts to spin their study results in published articles; with their failure to provide comprehensive, objective drug information in package inserts and the *PDR;* and with their use of drug advertising, sales representatives, and biased meetings and conferences to influence physicians. If doctors aren't properly informed, how can they properly select drugs for patients? And if patients aren't properly informed, how can they protect themselves?

Influence on Consumers

Drug-company efforts to influence consumers are equally effective—and of equal concern.

"People feel like the TV ads have convinced them that this medication will cure them forever, and they are reluctant to listen to other advice," Dr. Bradford Pontz told correspondent Jackie Judd of ABC News for her January 2001 report, "Truth in Advertising? FDA Says Many Prescription Drug Ads Are Deceptive."[103]

"They are leaving an impression on people's minds—and this is intentional—that the drugs can deliver more than they actually do," added Dr. Sharon Levine of Rx Alliance.[104]

Many people think that the FDA must approve television advertisements of medications beforehand, and that the advertised drugs must be completely safe. This isn't the case. "There is no guarantee that it's a balanced presentation or there is not some misleading information," the FDA's Tom Abrams told Judd.[105]

It is only after ads run that the understaffed FDA reviews them. Not surprisingly, the FDA has had to warn drug companies about making false claims, overstating the benefits of advertised drugs, making inaccurate safety claims, and minimizing the risks of side effects.[106] Each year the FDA has sent about one hundred letters to drug companies demanding changes in television commercials, magazine ads, and other promotional material.[107] The manufacturers of Celebrex have been cited three times, most recently for implying that the drug is more effective than demonstrated. Schering, the manufacturer of Claritin, has been cited ten times since 1997. Others cited include Lipitor, Prilosec, and Meridia.[108]

In 1999, Bayer aired a television advertisement for its aspirin. The advertising claimed that a small dose of aspirin daily would help prevent heart attacks. This is true—but this has been proven only for people with diagnosed cardiovascular disease. Yet, the advertisement glossed over this key point, leaving the impression that almost anyone might benefit from taking an aspirin every day.[109]

Most people aren't familiar with aspirin's limitations and dangers, and many people don't check with their physicians before starting over-the-counter drugs. Most people don't know that even small doses of aspirin can cause gastrointestinal bleeding. Gastrointestinal hemorrhaging occurs 80 percent more often in people taking low-dose aspirin.[110] Many people don't know that even small doses of aspirin can adversely affect kidney function and that aspirin increases the occurrence of strokes in people with high blood pressure.[111] The blood-thinning effects of aspirin can also increase bleeding from minor mishaps or cause increased bruising from injuries.

Unless a person has vascular disease, there are few reasons to take daily aspirin. But Bayer's ad was targeted directly to consumers, who are usually unaware of the downside. The FDA notified Bayer that it had to be changed, but the Bayer ad had already run.[112]

The FDA's ability to enforce advertising guidelines is limited. As of early 2001, it had not taken a single manufacturer to court. According to *Dickinson's FDA Review,* drug companies aren't concerned about receiving warning letters from the FDA,[113] because they face no significant penalties. There is, therefore, little to lose by stepping over the line. The drug-company attitude, according to William Vodra, former FDA associate chief counsel for drugs, is, "What will happen to me if I do [make false claims]?"[114] Usually the FDA sends a belated letter of reprimand, telling the company to change the advertisement. Of course, the advertisement has already run and exerted its intended influence.

Vodra told of drug companies that had gone to the FDA with complaints about competitors' unfair advertising and, according to *Dick-*

inson's FDA Review, "received verbal assurances of FDA intervention, only to see months go by without FDA action."[115] Thus, it is not surprising that direct-to-consumer prescription drug advertising is expected to increase to $7.5 billion by 2005, a 1,200% increase over a decade,[116] as drug manufacturers decide, as Vodra put it, to "fight fire with fire in the marketplace. It's only a small step from that to the adoption of an 'offense is the best defense' policy as marketing pressures intensify."[117]

Just Business

Should we be surprised by the actions of drug companies to slant their research favorably and to exert questionable influences on physicians and consumers? After all, drug companies are businesses, and as some economists assert, "The one and only social responsibility of business is to increase profits."

One can argue whether using unprincipled means to increase profits is socially responsible behavior. But if the reality is that maximum profits is the predominant ethos of the business world, then all of the drug-company policies described in this book make sense—that is, from a business point of view.

But the drug industry is unlike most other businesses. Drug companies aren't manufacturing toaster ovens or sunglasses, but extremely potent chemicals that people—medically ill people—require. Minor deviations from medical principles can cause widespread harm. I agree with Dr. Catherine DeAngelis, the editor in chief of *JAMA*, who in 2000 wrote: "Using business ethics without tempering them with the needs of society simply is not working."[118]

The situation has evolved to its current, unsatisfactory state for another reason. More than other industries, the drug companies are granted tremendous leeway because they produce vital products. The benefits of drug research are apparent to everyone. The drugs that have been developed over the last century have changed medical history and improved human health and longevity beyond even the imaginations of Jules Verne and H. G. Wells. Medical research has been one of humankind's greatest accomplishments. Yet, "research" is frequently invoked as the excuse for questionable drug-company actions and excessive profit-taking. Indeed, a decade ago, when the public image of the drug companies was faltering, the pharmaceutical industry adopted a public-relations strategy that emphasized its research. It was then that the drug companies added the word *research* to the name of their umbrella organization, the Pharmaceutical Research and Manufacturers of America (PhRMA).[119]

But even here, of the billions the drug industry devotes to research, a great deal is wasted on drugs that are developed not to provide new or better treatments for patients, but merely to grab a piece of a competitor's market. According to Dr. David Kessler, then the commissioner of the FDA, of the 127 new drugs produced between 1989 and 1993, "only a minority offered a clear clinical advantage over existing therapies."[120] Instead, Kessler and other FDA officials wrote:

> In today's prescription-drug marketplace, a host of similar products compete for essentially the same population of patients. . . .
> The preponderance of "me too" drugs has created a highly competitive marketplace for prescription drugs. Pharmaceutical companies are waging aggressive campaigns to change prescribers' habits and to distinguish their products from competing ones, even when the products are virtually indistinguishable. . . . Victory in these therapeutic-class wars can mean millions of dollars for a drug company. But for patients and providers it can mean misleading promotions, conflicts of interest, increased costs for health care, and ultimately, inappropriate prescribing.[121]

We can only wonder how many better and safer drugs might be available if the drug companies dedicated the bulk of their research budgets to discovering and developing truly useful new pharmaceuticals.

Of course, rather than impeding research, requiring drug companies to conduct scientifically sound research and more accurate marketing would improve drug safety. Setting some reasonable limits on promotional activities and advertising is also warranted and would free more funds for research. In her second 2000 article in *The New England Journal of Medicine*—"The Pharmaceutical Industry: To Whom Is It Accountable?"—then editor in chief Dr. Marcia Angell wrote, "The marketing budgets of the drug industry are enormous—much larger than the research and development costs. In 1999, Pfizer and Pharmacia & Upjohn spent nearly 40% of revenues on marketing and advertising."[122]

But don't expect the pharmaceutical industry to enact any reforms voluntarily, for they are fulfilling their business ethic—making profits—better than any other industry. The drug industry has been the most profitable industry in America over the last decade. According to Dr. Angell, American drug companies recorded a 21-percent increase in profits in 1999 alone. While other industries earned healthy profits averaging up to 12 percent annually over recent years, the drug industry has averaged 18.6 percent. Some drug companies' profits have approached 30 percent. At the same time, the drug companies have paid much lower taxes on their profits than many other industries.[123]

Prospects for continued high profits are excellent, because prices keep rising not only for new drugs, but by large increases in the costs of older medications that have long before covered the expenses of their research and development. The cost of drugs is the fastest-growing component of the health-care system, and nationwide it will soon exceed the costs of all physicians' fees. Already, at some HMOs, drug costs exceed the costs of all hospitalizations.[124] As hospitals and insurers shift more money to cover high drug prices, this means higher insurance premiums, fewer covered benefits, and higher co-payments for medical services and medications. Meanwhile, millions of people cannot afford vital medications, and as documented on television and in newspaper articles, seniors and other hard-pressed patients must travel to Canada or Mexico in order to obtain their medications at more affordable prices. Others go without.

Perhaps this would be different if people were able to purchase medications in the same manner in which they buy other products.

However, with prescription drug prices, market economics do not work, because the medication market is not open. When people purchase prescription drugs, it usually is not out of convenience but necessity. Getting a prescription isn't the same as shopping for a new suit or car. If someone is sick or in pain, obtaining treatment isn't elective. When people visit their physicians, it isn't just because they feel like shopping around for medications: It's because they need help. When a doctor prescribes a medication, the patient isn't likely to disagree or to even ask about the price. People don't usually quiz their doctors for cost comparisons (most doctors have no idea anyway), and people can't bargain with their pharmacists.

So, although patients are paying the tab and taking all of the risks, they are a captive audience. By requiring medication now and by having to purchase the specific drug doctors prescribe at the prices set by pharmacies, people are not operating in a free market as we know it. Of course, they can refuse the medication, but realistically, most of the time they really can't. Generic drugs, when available, can reduce costs substantially, but brand-name drugs receive patent protections lasting at least seventeen years. By that time, newer and better brand-name drugs have been developed that often make generic drugs second choices at best. For example, although generic ibuprofen is cheaper than Motrin, its brand-name predecessor, the development of Celebrex and Vioxx make these new, better, more expensive drugs the first choices for millions of patients.

Without an open market, consumers don't have freedom of choice. They cannot vote with their wallets. Doctors have choices, which drug companies vie to influence by producing drugs with higher, more impressive doses and simplistic, easy-to-use dosage guidelines. Once doctors select medications and write prescriptions, patients are as limited as soldiers with orders. They either follow them or suffer the consequences.

The result, as captured by Dr. Angell: "Once a drug is patented, no one else may sell it, and the drug company is free to charge whatever the traffic will bear."[125] This is why Viagra costs $9.50 a pop, and why the prices of other new drugs aren't far behind. This is why even for older drugs, drug companies can keep raising prices although these drugs' research was finished and paid for a decade ago. This is why a one-month, thirty-pill prescription for Claritin costs about $70. But when its patent finally expires, experts expect the cost of generic Claritin, loratadine, to cost about $20.

Perhaps we can't expect drug companies to act like charitable organizations. The pharmaceutical industry, like most industries, is profit-driven, and this drive is vital to the rapid development of important new drugs. However, it isn't unreasonable to expect reasonable drug prices that provide fair, not excessive, compensation to drug companies. It isn't unreasonable to expect the drug companies to provide properly tested drugs with dosages that fit people. It isn't unreasonable to expect the publication of all research results, unfavorable as well as favorable, so that new drugs can be evaluated fairly by physicians and consumers. It isn't unfair to expect reasonably accurate side-effect information and adequate warnings when new drugs are introduced, rather than after hundreds or thousands of people have been harmed.

Side Effects: Inevitable or Avoidable?

Most destructive of all, drug companies have been able to convince doctors and patients that side effects are unavoidable. Drug companies maintain that side effects are "inevitable," as I have heard their representatives say. This, it is explained, is because people differ so much in their responses to drugs. They are correct in one respect: people do differ a great deal. Beyond that, they are spinning the usual drug-industry line. The fact is, side effects are not inevitable. As we have seen, most side effects are the result of the known, dose-related actions of drugs in people who are being overmedicated. Proper doses—doses designed for people—avoid side effects. If you start low and increase slowly, most side effects never occur.

Individual variation has been an accepted medical principle for decades. When it is obeyed, drug therapy usually goes very well. Millions of people experience dose-related side effects and a hundred thousand die not because of individual variation, and not because side effects are inevitable, but because drug companies put too much money into marketing and too little into research, because they omit vital dosage studies and ignore individual variation, and because they do not design drugs to accommodate the differences between people.

The drug companies insist that tailoring drugs to fit people is impossible or financially impractical. This is false. Other industries not only recognize the differences among people, they capitalize on it. They produce cars, clothes, cosmetics, and hundreds of other commodities in vast arrays to match individual sizes and needs. If we have the ingenuity to do this in so many areas, are we supposed to believe that it cannot be accomplished with vital medications?

Considerable evidence proves that we can. Thyroid medications are made in eleven sizes, all scored, to facilitate precise dosing. Digoxin is carefully matched to the needs and tolerances of patients. Diabetics receive the same careful dosing with insulin. With these drugs, anything less than careful dose titration is considered negligent. Why not with all prescription drugs? In fact, a small number of specialists do prescribe antihypertensive drugs with similar "Start low, go slow" precision. I did the same with Prozac, Elavil, Valium, Xanax, antihistamines, sleep remedies, seizure medications, and other drugs that can cause many side effects. Once I ignored the drug companies' guidelines and took the time to individualize my patients' dosages, side effects were few and mild.

It can be done.

How Drug Companies Influence Drug Research and the Information Provided to Doctors and Patients

1. Favorably designed studies: Drug-company funded studies provide more favorable results regarding the company's drugs than the results obtained in studies conducted without drug-company funding.

2. Favorable Comparisons: Drug companies compare full dosages of their drugs to inadequate dosages of competing drugs or to older, less effective drugs. This makes their drugs appear superior even when they actually aren't.

3. Nonrepresentative new-drug studies: Testing is conducted with mostly young, healthy subjects rather than with older subjects, even if the new drug will be used primarily by older patients. Young subjects usually report better rates of improvement and fewer side effects. This provides more impressive yet misleading data for marketing the new drug.

4. Manipulating the measurement of effectiveness: Drug companies can employ several measures of effectiveness, then pick and choose the most favorable measures while suppressing the unfavorable findings. The new drug is then promoted with a misleadingly positive profile.

5. Publication of only favorable studies: Drug companies can pick and choose among multiple studies, publishing only the most favorable ones. They can design studies to obtain better outcomes and can avoid doing important studies that may reveal unfavorable results.

6. Suppression of vital information: If a study's results aren't to a drug company's liking, it can suppress the data or impede its publication. It can also keep studies from public awareness by declaring them "proprietary information." Researchers determined to publish important side-effect warnings may be threatened with lawsuits or loss of research funding.

7. Stacking data: A small amount of favorable data about a drug can be exaggerated by repackaging the information in different studies by different authors in different journals, creating the impression that the favorable data are considerable.

8. Spinning studies favorably: Contrary to ethical standards, drug companies hire ghostwriters who were not involved in studies to write favorable articles according to the companies' specifications. Drug companies also hire prestigious doctors to give drug studies status by fronting as authors of research articles, although the doctors played no role in the research.

9. Slanted symposia: Speakers at meetings sponsored by drug companies are chosen to present the companies' products favorably and to deemphasize side effects and other problems.

11. Misleading advertising: Drug companies can promote drugs through misleading advertising, and they can continue advertising questionable results even after independent studies reveal deficiencies and inaccuracies in these results.

Chapter 10

What the Drug Companies Must Do to Reverse the Side-Effect Epidemic— But Will They?

COMPETITION WITHIN the pharmaceutical industry has always been stiff, and it has impelled the development of beneficial new discoveries as well as unsafe drugs and improper marketing strategies. Harmful products with absurd claims necessitated the creation of the FDA in the early twentieth century. This brought many improvements, but not enough, for mounting competitive pressures have resulted in the production of a record number of new drugs requiring withdrawal and a new wave of questionable marketing techniques.

"The competitive pressures in the pharmaceutical marketplace are reaching new heights of intensity," according to *Dickinson's FDA Review.*[1] Market competition is, of course, a powerful drive, but market forces do not always reward quality or safety. With medications, marketing a new type of drug quickly is often more advantageous than taking extra time to conduct thorough research. Making dosages easy to use rather than fitting them to patients makes medications more popular with physicians. The marketplace may sometimes reward quality and safety, but it frequently rewards expediency and misrepresentation—in other words, shrewd marketing.

Corporations are self-perpetuating engines of economic activity and, therefore, are committed to shrewd marketing. No one person is in control. No one person is responsible. This is the advantage of corporations—and the danger, especially if the sole corporate ethic is to increase profits. Drug companies that get their products to market first can thrive even if their research is shoddy, their data is questionable, their articles are ghostwritten, and their dosage and side-effect information is inadequate.

Moreover, if a drug company's profits increase because of slanted research, hasty marketing, and misleading advertising, other companies must adopt these same methods in order to remain competitive—and the race to the bottom accelerates. This is why in any area of endeavor, codes of behavior must be periodically reexamined. Doing so is a common occurrence in politics and sports, and it is what the drug companies must now undertake.

"Reforms Required in Drug Company Research and Development" (see box section) lists several improvements in the early research of new medications that would greatly diminish side effects, improve patient satisfaction, and keep people in necessary treatment. One of these improvements would be for drug companies to list all studies before they begin with a neutral registry. For years, experts in Europe and the United States have sought this, thereby making all study results—favorable and unfavorable—available. By registering all studies beforehand, drug companies wouldn't be able to hide studies that proved to be unfavorable.

Previous efforts to create a volunteer drug research registry were unsuccessful. Some drug companies such as Schering and Glaxo Wellcome joined, but many did not. However, in 2001, Britain took a step toward the full disclosure of all drug studies. Since January 2001, the public can have access to a database of all clinical trials of new drugs in the United Kingdom (www.controlled-trials.com). Developed by the Association of the British Pharmaceutical Industry, it will provide immediate information about thousands of drug trials conducted annually in that country.

However, the impact of registering drug-company studies on improving drug safety will be small if the quality of the published information remains suspect. If the drug companies continue to influence how medication studies are designed, performed, analyzed, and published, the low quality of information that physicians receive will continue to foster unnecessary risks for patients. Thus, Dr. Marcia Angell, the former editor in chief of *The New England Journal of Medicine*, commented, "I have no quarrel with drug companies funding research, only with the terms. There should be no strings attached."[2]

But expecting drug companies to desist from influencing studies is unrealistic. With huge sums and careers at stake, the incentive to design studies and interpret results in the most favorable manner will remain—and sometimes be too tempting to resist. Doctors hired by drug companies cannot avoid conflicts of interests in performing their research. Drug companies geared to satisfying the limited FDA requirements for drug approval will not invest the extra time and money for conducting research that is comprehensive enough to address the diverse issues that arise when doctors prescribe a new drug to millions of patients.

This is why a national center for independent drug testing, as Dr. Raymond Woosley has suggested (Chapter 9), is necessary. Because of the demands of the marketplace for speed, drug companies will not conduct many important studies. Because the FDA requires drug companies to prove only that a new drug works for one specific condition, drug companies will often forgo studying other conditions for which the same drug may be effective. These gaps in drug research could be filled by an independent national drug research center funded by a pool of federal, private, and pharmaceutical-industry money.

The studies conducted at an independent research center could be better designed and more applicable to the everyday needs of doctors and patients. Such studies could also obtain more accurate side-effect profiles of medications. Independent researchers would have no conflicts of interest and no conscious or subconscious motive for missing side effects or minimizing their importance.

An independent research center could study other uses of new medications that were not studied by their manufacturers. It could research new uses or problems with generic drugs, which drug companies do not study because the patents of generic drugs have lapsed and there is little likelihood of profit.

Even if the pharmaceutical industry undertakes proper self-regulation or if public pressure leads to improved government regulation, the need for objective information will remain. A national medication research center is a good investment, because confirming the effectiveness of medications and determining the true extent of side effects will improve drug safety and usage in America. In doing so, it will save lives and reduce long-term health-care costs.

PERHAPS THE MOST significant improvement that drug companies must enact is the routine determination of the lowest, safest effective doses of all medications and the publication of this information in all package inserts and *PDR* descriptions. Defining the lowest, safest, most effective dosages isn't difficult. It doesn't require longer or additional studies. It can be accomplished by simply adding a low-dosage group to studies that are already required for testing new drugs.

"The entire clinical experience during Phases 1 through 3 [of new drug research] should be the basis of dosing recommendations for individualized treatment," wrote Dr. Carl Peck, highly respected FDA officer Dr. Robert Temple, and fifteen other physicians. "The information derived therefore can be used . . . to help practitioners appreciate the existence of interpatient variability [differences between different patients] in response and its causes, and the way to avoid adverse drug experiences due to such variability. Wording in the label should be developed to communicate to prescribers . . . some appreciation of intrapatient [the differing needs of a patient at different times] and interpatient variability and its causes, so that they will be able to individualize treatment."[3]

The absurdity of the current system, which ignores effective low doses, is apparent when a decade after drug companies market their products, when some are approaching expiration of their patents, the companies decide that lower doses of these drugs would indeed be effective as over-the-counter products. Over-the-counter Motrin, Orudis, Aleve, Pepcid, Axid, Tagamet, Zantac, and some antihistamines all began as higher-dose prescription drugs. In the years before these lower, over-the-counter doses became available, people going to their physicians with the same mild disorders were prescribed higher doses—doses often 100 percent higher than they now get with these same medications at lower over-the-counter doses. In other words, even though it may have been evident for years that lower, safer doses of Motrin, Tagamet, and these other drugs worked, their manufacturers did not recommend these lower doses—until the time was ripe for marketing them as low-dose, over-the-counter products.

Actually, with Zantac, a top-selling drug in the U.S. for many years in the 1980's, the package insert did advise doctors about a lower effective dosage. The standard Zantac dosage was 150 mg twice daily, but the Zantac package insert and *PDR* description stated, "Smaller doses have been shown to be equally effective in inhibiting gastric acid secretion in US studies, and several foreign trials have shown that 100 twice-daily is as effective as the 150-mg dose [twice daily]." Yet, although I asked many physicians and pharmacists, I never found one who had noticed this lower dose. It wouldn't have mattered, because the smallest Zantac pill at that time was 150 mg. In 1996, Zantac finally became available in a lower dose as over-the-counter Zantac-75, which contains 75 mg, a dose sufficient for mild cases.

The same process is evident in 2001. For example, an impressive study has shown that a lower dosage of Celebrex,[4] the top-selling anti-inflammatory drug, is effective and causes fewer side effects than the doses currently recommended by Searle. This lower dose of Celebrex (50 mg twice daily) is 50 percent lower than the lowest prescription dosage (100 mg twice daily) available today, but the smallest pill that Searle makes is a 100-mg capsule. However, years from now, perhaps when it serves the company's goals, Searle may decide that low-dose Celebrex is indeed effective and worthy of over-the-counter production. This strategy has already been enacted with Motrin, Aleve, and Orudis. When low-dose Celebrex is finally made available as an over-the-counter drug, consumers will at last have access to a lower, safer dosage that was proven to work in 1999. But until Searle decides the production of low-dose Celebrex serves its corporate purposes, many people will continue receiving higher doses of Celebrex than they need, and they will continue being exposed to heightened risks of gastrointestinal bleeding, kidney damage, and other dose-related side effects.

Marketing strategies should not determine when a lower, safer drug dosage should be manufactured. It should be manufactured from the start.

CLARITIN AND ALLEGRA, popular prescription antihistamines, provide a different type of example. Whereas Claritin and Allegra represent a second generation of antihistamines that infrequently cause drowsiness, all of the over-the-counter antihistamines available today are first-generation antihistamines that are notorious for causing drowsiness in as many as 50 percent of users. Indeed, one of the doses of over-the-counter Benadryl and generic diphenhydramine that is recommended for daytime allergy relief is also recommended in Nytol, Unisom, Sleep-eze, and Sominex for promoting sleep. Therefore, it is not surprising that over-the-counter drugs that sedate people have been linked to automobile accidents and fatalities.[5] Replacing the older, side-effect-prone, over-the-counter antihistamines with Claritin and Allegra would save lives.

In fact, in a March 2000 study in the *Annals of Internal Medicine*, people's driving abilities were tested after being given over-the-counter Benadryl, prescription Allegra, alcohol, or a placebo. The effects of Allegra and the placebo were similar. Not surprisingly, alcohol at a blood concentration of 0.1 percent—legal intoxication in many states—impaired driving ability. But over-the-counter Benadryl, as the researchers wrote, "had a greater impact on driving than alcohol did."[6]

Instead of waiting for years for the most profitable moment for manufacturing low-dose, over-the-counter Allegra and Claritin, these drugs should be made available as soon as possible, so that people have other options instead of highly sedating over-the-counter antihistamines like Benadryl. This was also the conclusion of a federal commission that in May 2001 reviewed a petition for making Allegra, Claritin, and Zyrtec available over-the-counter, despite the opposition of their manufacturers. However, while the medical basis for making Claritin and Allegra over-the-counter seems clear, the financial aspects aren't simple. These drugs represent major investments and important sources of income for their manufacturers. Claritin is Schering's largest earner, allowing the company to remain competitive with larger rivals. The pharmaceutical industry and government must develop a process by which newer, better over-the-counter drugs can be brought to market as soon as their advantages over current products are evident. In return, a method of compensating manufacturers needs to be created.

LISTING THE REFORMS needed in drug-company policies is the easy part. The hard part is to get the drug companies to enact them. The pharmaceutical industry is enjoying great financial success; can it be convinced nonetheless that changes are imperative in order to improve medical care and drug safety? Can the pharmaceutical industry even admit some of its excesses?

Actually, the drug companies should want to improve their methods, because they, too, would benefit where it most counts for them: the bottom line. What good does it do the drug companies when 50 percent of patients placed on medications for serious conditions such as elevated cholesterol or high blood pressure quit treatment? What good does it do the drug companies when people are afraid to fill prescriptions, and when tens of millions would rather try unregulated, unproven, haphazardly manufactured herbal supplements rather than regulated and proven medications?

Improved safety would increase medication usage. Treating patients like individuals would produce fewer side effects, better results, greater satisfaction for patients and physicians, and greater overall confidence in the medical system. Millions of people who now turn to unproven, unregulated alternative remedies might realize the preferability of pharmaceuticals that are proven effective, reliably produced, government-regulated, and safely dosed. These improvements would lead to less bad publicity, more sales, and more profits.

I like to think that drug-company employees would also feel better about themselves and their accomplishments. I cannot believe that they are pleased with the continued high incidence of side effects and the almost daily stories about newly discovered dangers with their products. They cannot be happy with the record number of FDA withdrawals and the growing suspicion among consumers that the drug industry cannot be trusted to produce safe products. Drug-company executives must realize that people are losing confidence in the system upon which the drug companies' continuing success depends. Perhaps the pharmaceutical industry believes that the breakthroughs in genetics will lead to drugs that will keep the money flowing, but if the side-effect epidemic continues and consumer confidence continues to sag, as much will be lost as gained.

Most difficult, how do you get all of the drug companies to agree? Some drug-company officials already recognize these problems and are unsatisfied with the current situation, but unilateral adherence to the recommendations listed here would be suicidal for any one company. The pharmaceutical industry needs a Geneva agreement, a code of acceptable behavior that provides a better balance between marketing and medical science.

Regrettably, the history of voluntary compliance among corporations is not encouraging. Automobile companies did not add seat belts willingly. Cigarette companies did not add warnings willingly. American industry did not embrace environmental protection willingly.

Without adequate self-regulation, the activities of the drug companies require external oversight and regulation. The regulatory agency overseeing the pharmaceutical industry is the Food and Drug Administration. But how effective is the FDA in controlling drug-company activities? As discussed in Chapter 9, the FDA has little control over drug-company advertising and little power to ensure that drug companies complete studies agreed upon as a condition for approval of many new drugs. The FDA is supposed to ensure that new drugs are safe and effective, but since 1997 more drugs have been withdrawn because of toxicities than ever before. How well is the FDA overseeing the drug companies? How well is it ensuring drug safety? In the next chapter, we will examine these questions.

Reforms Required in Drug-Company Research, Development, and Marketing

1. Define and manufacture the very lowest effective doses of new drugs. Unless medical or chemical factors require otherwise, medications should be made as scored tablets in several dose sizes.

2. Test new drugs against the most effective drugs currently used for the same indications. Drugs should be compared at equivalent doses.

3. Register all studies at the time they are begun with a centralized, neutral registry.

4. Publish all study results, favorable and unfavorable, promptly. Disclose all direct and indirect drug-company involvement in studies.

5. Limit involvement in drug studies to funding and general design. Drug companies should have no involvement in specific drug-study design, analysis, or publishing of results: These should be left to the researchers.

6. The authors of published studies should have direct involvement in designing or conducting the drug studies. No ghostwriters or ghost authors. No influencing authors or shaping their comments.

7. The drug companies and the FDA must utilize measures of effectiveness that do not produce unnecessarily high doses. Effectiveness must be defined and proven in ways that reflect the actual needs of patients.

8. The use of "proprietary rights" for withholding information should not extend to the suppression of important drug information or side effects.

9. New drugs with potential risks should be approved conditionally, with limited and specific uses, and should be closely monitored until safety is assured.

10. Package inserts and *PDR* descriptions should provide current, comprehensive dose-response and side-effect information.

11. Dosage guidelines should define the broad range of individual variation among patients and that side effects and long-term risks are minimized by using the lowest, safest doses required for each person.

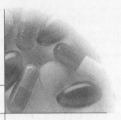

Chapter 11

What's Wrong with the FDA? And What Can Be Done About It?

THROUGH ALL OF THESE chapters you have probably been wondering, "Why isn't the FDA doing more about these problems?" Most Americans think of the FDA as a watchdog agency, but in recent years the watchdog has shown less bark and bite.

"Do I have less confidence in the drug approval process? Absolutely," Dr. Lisa McCoy, a family practitioner in Ashland, Kentucky, told the *Los Angeles Times*."[1] In 1997, McCoy, like many physicians, had great hopes for a newly approved diabetes drug, Rezulin. So did the thousands of patients whose diabetes was poorly controlled by the other diabetes drugs already available.

So did Warner-Lambert, Rezulin's manufacturer, which as early as 1995 was making sure that Rezulin was well-received not only by doctors, but by the investment community. According to a series of indepth articles in the *Los Angeles Times* that earned a Pulitzer Prize for reporter David Willman, Warner-Lambert had launched an extensive marketing campaign long before Rezulin was approved by the FDA.

The campaign included pitches to Wall Street analysts emphasizing the drug's potential market of over fifteen million Americans with adult-onset diabetes.[2] The company or its affiliates paid fees to hundreds of doctors for speaking about the promising new drug. It paid for free travel to the 1996 Olympic games for diabetes specialists, who by prescribing Rezulin could make it a billion-dollar drug.[3] Yet, the medical officers at the FDA hadn't even finished their analysis of the Rezulin data.

In fact, the FDA officer in charge of evaluating Rezulin, Dr. John Gueriguian, wasn't so sanguine about Rezulin. Compared to approved oral medications for diabetes, Rezulin "offered very little significant advantage," according to a summary of an FDA meeting in the summer of 1996.[4] A few months later, Gueriguian, a veteran of many drug evaluations, concluded, according to the *Times,* "that Rezulin was unfit for approval and warned of its potential to harm the liver and the heart."[5] Warner-Lambert executives protested. Gueriguian was relieved from the evaluation of Rezulin, and the FDA approved Rezulin for general usage in the spring of 1997.[6,7]

Rezulin did help some people who hadn't done well on other diabetes remedies. "Rezulin worked and it worked great," Dr. McCoy said after prescribing it to about a dozen patients.[8] But in October 1997, just a few months after approving Rezulin, the FDA received the first cases of severe liver failure related to the drug. One FDA officer, Dr. Robert Misbin, recorded in his diary, "We have real trouble." Misbin reexamined Warner-Lambert's original research and the recent case reports and concluded that the FDA "knew the essential truth—that Rezulin could cause liver failure. There was a potential for disaster."[9]

The key question was: Did the good that Rezulin was doing for some patients outweigh the harm occurring in others? This wasn't easy to gauge. If Rezulin helped some people more than other diabetes drugs, how much more in terms of controlling these patients' diabetes and in preventing long-term consequences such as blindness, nerve injuries, limb amputations, and premature deaths? How could these benefits be weighed against the infrequent but serious cases of jaundice, weakness, and liver failure caused by Rezulin?

These questions didn't remain unanswered for long. Weighing a drug's major benefits against some minor if unpleasant side effects is one thing. Weighing these benefits against disabling, lethal side effects is another. In fact, in December 1997, following the disclosure of six Rezulin-related deaths, British regulatory officials withdrew Rezulin from use in Britain.[10,11]

But the FDA, despite the misgivings of Gueriguian and Misbin, did not follow Britain's example. For years Congress, which controls the FDA's funding, had been pressuring the FDA to cut in half the usual two-year process of approving new drugs. Finally, Congress enacted legislation that reduced the FDA's funding while mandating a fast-track approval process. The FDA got the message and made Rezulin its first "fast-track" diabetes drug. After evaluating Rezulin for only six months, the FDA announced its approval in early 1997. Before the year was out, Rezulin was banned in Britain, but not in the United States.

Rezulin's staunchest proponent at the FDA was Dr. Murray Lumpkin, who had prior ties to the drug industry as a director of international research for Abbott Laboratories.[12,13] At the FDA, Dr. Lumpkin was the deputy director of the drug evaluation center, and he had overseen the rapid approval of Rezulin and overruled Gueriguian's and Misbin's misgivings. Now, with the reports of Rezulin-related liver toxicities and deaths, Lumpkin and other FDA supporters of the drug required Warner-Lambert to add new warnings to Rezulin's labeling.[14]

Previously in this book I described the inadequacy and ineffectiveness of labeling changes with Seldane, women's hormones, and other drugs. For years, experts have challenged the FDA's reliance on warning labels to protect patients. The fact is, doctors don't keep rereading the package labels or *PDR* descriptions of drugs they've prescribed many times. The ineffectiveness of FDA-mandated labeling changes was underscored again in an article titled "Drug Labeling Revisions— Guaranteed to Fail?" by Dr. Raymond Woosley in a December 2000 issue of *JAMA*.[15]

It wasn't surprising, therefore, that the series of four labeling changes that Warner-Lambert added for Rezulin accomplished little—except it did allow Warner-Lambert to keep Rezulin on the market an additional twenty-seven months. During this time, the company earned $1.8 billion.[16]

The initial labeling changes advised doctors to monitor the liver functioning of patients taking Rezulin. When this proved inadequate, the next labeling changes recommended more liver tests more frequently. Yet, there was never any proof that such testing would adequately protect patients, as Dr. Janet Woodcock, director of the FDA drug evaluation center, later knowledged.[17,18] In fact, Rezulin liver toxicity could occur very quickly. In the months between blood tests, a Rezulin user could develop liver damage of major, even lethal proportions. This was seen when Audrey LaRue Jones, a 55-year-old teacher, died of liver failure on May 17, 1998. Jones was a volunteer in a Rezulin study sponsored jointly by Warner-Lambert and the National Institutes of Health.[19] If the close monitoring of the NIH couldn't protect patients taking Rezulin, what could?

If Dr. Lumpkin and other FDA officials had believed that relying upon regular liver tests would protect patients, Jones's death should have changed their minds. So should have the death of Rosa Delia Valenzuela, a healthy 63-year-old woman—and the wife of famed jockey Ismael Valenzuela—who developed liver failure within a month of starting Rezulin in a closely monitored program.[20] Still, it took more than another year after Jones's and Valenzuela's deaths for the FDA to shift its stance, and even then it took a virtual revolt by mid-level FDA officers to force top officials to act.

One of the FDA physicians pressing for Rezulin's removal was Dr. David Graham. His startling analysis in early 1999 revealed:

- At least 430 people had already suffered liver failure with Rezulin.
- The risk of developing liver failure increased 1,200 percent in patients placed on Rezulin.
- One patient out of every 1,800 taking Rezulin would develop liver failure.[21]

Whereas Warner-Lambert had claimed that liver failure occurred only in one in 100,000 patients—a worrisome number in itself—Graham's findings showed that the actual incidence was fifty-five times greater. Moreover, Graham found that regular testing offered no guarantee of safety, because liver damage with Rezulin could occur so quickly and unpredictably.[22]

These findings challenged the accuracy of Warner-Lambert's information on Rezulin. Dr. William L. Isley, a diabetes specialist in Kansas City, Mo., who was involved in the development of Rezulin, told the *Los Angeles Times*, "The drug never should have gotten to market. The whole thing is a travesty."[23]

Meanwhile, doctors continued writing millions of prescriptions for Rezulin. In 1999 they wrote more than five million prescriptions for the drug. These included hundreds of thousands of Rezulin prescriptions to new patients. Obviously the warning labels hadn't alerted doctors or patients sufficiently about the full extent of Rezulin's risks. The labels didn't mention that the drug had been withdrawn in Britain years earlier, and that cases of liver failure and death continued to be reported to the FDA.

When Dr. McCoy became aware of Rezulin's dangers, she warned all of her Rezulin patients. Most decided to quit the drug, but Dianna Barnett, who'd had difficulties with other diabetes drugs, decided to stay on Rezulin. Barnett, 56, worked as a home health aide and volunteered as a Sunday-school teacher. After doing very well on Rezulin for eighteen months under McCoy's close supervision, in June 1999 Barnett became gravely ill from acute liver failure. As of June 2000, the liver failure was causing severe fatigue, pain, and swelling, while Barnett awaited a liver transplant.[24]

"I feel horrible for her," Dr. McCoy said of Barnett. "All you want to do is do good for your patients, and with your best intentions something horrible like this happens." She added, "It's a real tragedy. We as physicians trust the FDA to give us good medications to use. We can't do the research ourselves."[25]

AFTER GRAHAM'S STARTLING analysis, it still took the FDA another year to act decisively. By February 2000, the FDA had confirmed 85 cases of liver failure and 58 deaths attributable to Rezulin.[26] But despite growing sentiment within the medical community for Rezulin's withdrawal—sentiments shared by experts such as Vanderbilt's Dr. Alastair Wood, who was the drug therapy editor for *The New England Journal of Medicine*, and the FDA's own Dr. Robert Temple[27]—FDA officials continued holding meetings with Warner-Lambert representatives. At one meeting, Misbin and Temple challenged the company's claim that liver monitoring worked. Misbin asked them, "How many more unnecessary deaths will it take before you take action?"[28]

On March 21, 2000, Janet Woodcock, Lumpkin, Misbin, Graham, Temple, and a dozen other FDA specialists met again. Graham estimated that twenty more cases of liver failure would occur each succeeding month that Rezulin remained available.[29] After further deliberations, the FDA announced that it would ask Warner-Lambert to withdraw Rezulin. By this time the FDA had confirmed sixty-three deaths from Rezulin-related liver failures—and outside experts estimated the actual number to be five to ten times higher.[30]

WHAT HAD BEEN LEARNED from the Rezulin fiasco? Dr. McCoy felt betrayed by the FDA and now waits for more safety information before recommending any new drugs to her patients.[31]

Dr. Isley learned the same lesson after a patient of his died of liver failure from Rezulin: "The FDA used to serve a purpose. A doctor could feel sure that a drug he was prescribing was as safe as possible. Now you wonder what kind of evaluation has been done, and what's been swept under the rug."[32]

"They've lost their compass and they forgot who it is that they are ultimately serving," said Lemuel Moye, a University of Texas School of Public Health physician who served from 1995 to 1999 on an FDA advisory committee.[33]

Just as I had learned with Prozac, Xanax, and many other drugs a decade earlier, the Rezulin disaster taught many physicians that the current methods of the drug companies and the safety mechanisms of the FDA cannot be relied upon. They cannot be trusted to provide safe drugs or safe dosages. However, if every doctor has to learn this lesson drug tragedy by drug tragedy, such tragedies will never end, and the high incidence of medication-related reactions and deaths will continue.

Surprisingly, not everyone perceived the Rezulin experience negatively. Some high officials at the FDA saw it as proof that their system works. "I don't think the fact that a drug is taken off the market is an indication that it should not have been approved," Dr. John Jenkins, director of a drug evaluation office for the FDA, told *The New York Times*. "All drugs have risks. Some we don't learn about until after the drug is approved."[34]

But any good scientist knows that if a few cases of liver injury occur among a couple of thousand study subjects over a relatively short time frame, a much greater number including some that are severe will almost invariably occur when the drug is taken for years by millions of patients in the general population. An agency that is truly dedicated to the safety of patients recognizes this and avoids these possibilities rather than explaining away the risks.

Indeed, contradicting Jenkins's reasoning, an endocrinologist at UCLA who participated in the early testing of Rezulin told *The New York Times* that Rezulin's liver toxicity was obvious before it was approved.[35] Some liver tests were so abnormal that the dangers were obvious. According to a November 1997 FDA report, thirteen research patients had liver toxicity resulting in blood-enzyme levels more than ten times normal.[36] In five patients, the liver enzyme levels exceeded normal by thirty times. Yet, despite all of these warning signs, Warner-Lambert still didn't recommend liver testing for Rezulin users in its initial product information for doctors, and the FDA didn't require them.[37]

At a May 2000 meeting, Dr. Lumpkin defended the FDA's handling of Rezulin, but Dr. Jules Hirsch of Rockefeller University wasn't buying it. "I don't share the point of view of a wonderfully happy outcome, of how well the system has worked. A lot of people died of this thing. And a lot more people than we know died."[38]

WHAT'S GOING ON at the FDA? In August 2000, the watchdog group Public Citizen posted on its Web site the results of a survey of medical officers at the FDA. Their comments provided a portrait of a divided agency.

"My feeling after more than 20 years at the FDA is that unless drugs cannot be shown to 'kill patients' outright, then they will be approved with revised labeling and box warning," one medical officer wrote.

Another stated: "We are shifting the burden of proof of safety onto ourselves. Instead of asking the drug companies to prove the drug is safe, we are trying to prove the drug dangerous. If we cannot show that the drug is dangerous, then it is assumed safe."

Ninety-two percent of the FDA officers responding to the Public Citizen survey said that they were under increased pressure to approve drugs more quickly. "What are the options?" one wrote. "Everything must now be approved or approvable." Another commented, "The default seems to be 'yes' [to approval]; the hurdle to disapprove a drug is much higher than approving it."[39]

Even when medical officers decide a drug is unsafe, they are frequently overruled. A January 1999 Public Citizen reported that twenty-seven drugs had received FDA approval over the opposition of the medical officers in charge of the drugs. One officer wrote, "In the last two years, I recommended that two drugs not be approved. They were both approved without consulting me. This never happened before. In one case, the drug did not meet the standards set up by the division, so they nullified the standards." The officers described getting harassing telephone calls from drug-company representatives, receiving pressure from Congress to expedite drug approvals, and being prevented by their own superior officers from providing vital drug information to the decision-making committees.[40]

Distressed by the agency's policies, Dr. Misbin, a career FDA officer, put his career on the line when he sent a letter criticizing the new FDA policies to *The Washington Post*. "The more new drugs are approved, the more productive the FDA appears, even if the new drugs are not as good as what is available already."[41]

In a letter he posted on his Web site in late 2000, Dr. Robert Fenichel, a deputy division director at the FDA from 1996 to 2000, commented that at the FDA's higher levels, "the Agency keeps score by counting approvals."[42]

After its August 2000 survey, Public Citizen concluded, "Changes in the FDA review and approval process in the past several years appear to have led to a significant decline in the safety and efficacy standards for new drugs. These findings should raise a red flag that the very integrity of the drug-approval process in the United States, long an example to the rest of the world, is being seriously eroded."[43]

The February 1999 issue of *Dickinson's FDA Review* echoed Public Citizen's findings: "Many in the agency are uncomfortable with the aspects of a 'kinder, gentler FDA' that are seen as yielding too much to outside interests, especially regulated industry."[44]

WAS REZULIN an exception? Unfortunately not.

Lotronex was approved in early 2000. Within a month the FDA began receiving reports of severe reactions with the drug. After eight months, the numbers totaled ninety-three hospitalizations, multiple emergency bowel surgeries, and five deaths associated with Lotronex. By August 2000, the FDA responded—by requiring new warnings. Public Citizen disagreed: "It is irresponsible for Glaxo Wellcome and for the FDA to allow this doomed drug to stay on the market any longer."[45]

A *Los Angeles Times* investigation published in early November 2000 found: "FDA officials disregarded the significance of concerns raised by an agency medical officer who examined the drug before its approval."[46] A year earlier, in November 1999, Dr. John Senior, an FDA medical officer and bowel specialist, raised concerns about rushing Lotronex toward approval. In his review, Senior stated that it was "very disturbing that the applicant [Glaxo Wellcome] has chosen to downplay so strongly the important issue of constipation induced commonly and predictably, and has totally ignored the [problems] of ischemic colitis." Ischemic colitis results from a blockage of blood flow to the colon and can cause severe pain, permanent damage, and death. Senior added, "This finding represents a signal of a potentially serious problem."[47]

But the FDA approved Lotronex—and eleven months later, after the numbers of hospitalizations and deaths continued rising, it withdrew the drug in November 2000.

SUCH STORIES ARE not uncommon at today's FDA. Viagra was approved with inadequate warnings about easily anticipated problems in cardiac patients. The result? Hundreds died. Not only that, Viagra causes major interactions with several AIDS drugs, but although these interactions should have been foreseen, they weren't. It took over one and a half years before the PDR offered any warning to doctors and patients about these serious, life-threatening interactions. How many died unnecessarily? We'll never know.

Senior FDA officials also ignored warnings about the dangers of Posicor, a new drug for treating high blood pressure. "I sure don't feel good about what I've seen," said Dr. Lemuel Moye, a member of the FDA's Cardiovascular and Renal Drug Advisory Committee, on February 28, 1997. Dr. Moye suggested delaying the decision. Dr. Robert Califf, another advisory committee member, said, "If this [drug] was really something that was dramatically different, better than anything else in the way of relieving symptoms, then I would look at it differently. But given the fact that there are a lot of other effective therapies out there, why not be safe with the public?"[48]

In Sweden, authorities decided against approving Posicor.[49] In the U.S., Posicor was approved on June 20, 1997. After receiving reports of one hundred deaths following the drug's use, it was withdrawn on June 8, 1998.

Dr. Moye said, "Posicor should not have been approved. Therefore, any death that was attributable to Posicor was an unnecessary death."[50]

DID THE FDA tighten its approval standards after the Rezulin and Lotronex fiascoes? Apparently not. In April 2000, an FDA advisory committee approved a new drug for impotence: Uprima.[51] Actually, the chemical it contains, apomorphine, has been around a long time, but it causes so many side effects, its appropriateness for general usage was questionable. But after Viagra generated more than $1 billion in annual sales, apomorphine received another look. Besides, Uprima could be produced as a lozenge that, by dissolving in the mouth, would hit the bloodstream three times faster than Viagra—a great marketing advantage. TAP Pharmaceuticals applied for FDA approval of Uprima even though the drug was effective in only 25 percent more patients than placebo. It not only failed 40 percent of the time, but more than half of the study subjects quit because of side effects. Nausea occurred in 20 percent of Uprima users, dizziness in 14 percent, and a substantial, potentially dangerous drop in blood pressure in 3 percent.[52] Such side effects are usually dose-related.

During research studies, one patient took Uprima in his doctor's office and, when nothing untoward occurred, drove home—then blacked out and rammed his car into a fence.[53] Another study volunteer passed out and fractured his skull on his doctor's office floor. The FDA advisory committee recommended a highlighted box in the Uprima product information warning about some of Uprima's side effects. This fit the new FDA methodology as described by an agency medical officer in the Public Citizen survey: "We are in the midst now to approve everything but to describe drug weaknesses in the label."[54]

But not all members were supportive of the FDA's advisory-committee decision to approve Uprima. One panel member was so disturbed that he dissented publicly: "Some people will probably lose their lives because they pass out at the top of the stairs or operating a car. The complications that have been seen . . . are frightening."[55]

How could an FDA advisory committee approve Uprima—or Rezulin, or Lotronex—without adequate safeguards? Or Viagra without adequate warnings for cardiac patients? Aren't these committees, composed of experts from the medical community, supposed to provide a patient-oriented perspective on new drugs? According to a USA Today investigation, "More than half of the experts hired to advise the government on the safety and effectiveness of medicine have financial relationships with the pharmaceutical companies that will be helped or hurt by their decisions." Experts on advisory committees are supposed to be independent, but according to USA Today, "54% of the time, they have a direct financial interest in the drug or topic they are asked to evaluate. These conflicts include helping a pharmaceutical company develop a medicine, then serving on an FDA advisory committee that judges the drug."[56] On many committees, advisors with drug company ties outnumber independent advisors.

Federal law prevents government agencies from hiring experts with financial conflicts of interest, but since 1998 "the FDA has waived the restriction more than 800 times," *USA Today* found.[57] The problem involves hundreds of experts making decisions on drugs that will be taken by millions of Americans and that will earn billions of dollars for the drug industry. In the case of Rezulin, the *Los Angeles Times* found: "The manufacturer of the diabetes pill Rezulin provided fees or hefty research grants to at least a dozen scientists who also weighed the safety of the controversial drug for the federal government, records and interviews show."[58]

Dickinson's PDA Review commented in December 2000: "Advisory committee bias has been a recurring issue for the FDA over the years."[59] In June 2001, *The Washington Times* reported that a congressional committee was "investigating claims of mismanagement and influence peddling involving the committees that evaluate the safety and efficacy of new drugs."[60]

The looming controversy over Uprima ended for the moment in June 2000 when officials at TAP pharmaceuticals suspended its application pending further studies. Still, it was hardly reassuring that although the manufacturer itself finally recognized the potential problems with Uprima, the FDA advisory committee—which is supposed to place public safety first—did not.

In May 2001 Uprima received approval in Europe—at a lower dose.

THE FDA MAY also have missed problems associated with Herceptin. After usage in approximately 23,000 patients, this drug for breast cancer was already linked to fifteen deaths and sixty-two other severe hypersensitivity reactions.[61,62] Of course, reported reactions are usually just the tip of the iceberg, but using just the reported deaths, this amounts to an incidence of one death per fifteen hundred patients—an extremely high incidence. Preapproval studies are supposed to identify adverse reactions of this frequency, but somehow they weren't identified with Herceptin. The Herceptin package insert now contains a warning about these reactions.

Duract was similar to more than a dozen other anti-inflammatory medications already on the market except that, according to one FDA medical reviewer, it caused more liver toxicity than any of its competitors.[63] Yet, rather than deny Wyeth-Ayerst's application for this unnecessary drug, Duract was approved with a warning that it should be used for only ten days. Such warnings are as effective as producing a car that can go 150 miles per hour with a warning not to drive it over 35 mph. Human nature doesn't work that way, especially when advertising maximizes the benefits and minimizes the risks of medications. In his April 2000 article "The FDA In Crisis," Dr. Thomas J. Moore of George Washington University wrote: "So effective is the industry at marketing, and so uncritical are prescribing physicians, that more than 2.5 million prescriptions of Duract were written in the 10 months before Duract was withdrawn because of the expected, predictable, and entirely preventable liver deaths." Moore concluded, "The agency has accommodated industry by accepting risky drugs, and when these drugs triggered concerns, simply issued warnings to doctors rather than promptly removing the drugs from the market." Why is the FDA doing this? Moore answered: "In a push for quick approval for new drugs, the tilt to industry has gone too far."[64]

OTHER FDA DEFICIENCIES that harm patients are more subtle. As chapters 2 through 8 describe in detail, the FDA allows drug companies to market drugs at doses that overmedicate millions of people. Indeed, the FDA's own methods of evaluating effectiveness cause drug companies to develop drug doses that are higher than many people need. But none of this explains why the FDA approved Lilly's recommendation for starting all patients at 20 mg/day of Prozac even though a study had already been published demonstrating that just 5 mg was sufficient for 54 percent of patients. The FDA approved Lipitor and Celebrex at doses that are 100 percent higher than many people require. The FDA approved Prilosec, the best-selling drug in America in 1999, at an initial dose of 20 mg/day for everyone, even though 10 mg was sufficient for many ulcer patients.[65] Surely this lower dosage may be useful for older patients, Asian patients who metabolize the drug slowly, and mild cases of gastritis or heartburn. Indeed, similar dosage problems may have doomed Lotronex: Several people helped by the drug told *The New York Times* that they felt the dosage was too high. At least one person split the dosage for himself and obtained good results with fewer side effects.

Moreover, the FDA compounded these and scores of other mistakes by allowing manufacturers to omit their low-dosage information from package inserts and *PDR* descriptions. This has kept doctors and patients in the dark for decades about the effectiveness and greater safety of lower dosages. Thus, while the media has provided considerable attention to the harm caused by withdrawn drugs such as Rezulin, Lotronex, Duract, Fen-Phen, Redux, and others, it is the unrecognized approval of unnecessarily high drug dosages and the failure to inform physicians and patients about the effectiveness of lower, safer dosages that has fueled the greater part of the side-effect epidemic.

EVEN WHEN SOME new drugs help people, the FDA's policies have caused them harm too. In a January 2001 article in *The New York Times* titled "FDA Pulls a Drug, and Patients Despair," reporter Denise Grady described how the withdrawal of Lotronex affected some people:

> As soon as he learned that Lotronex was being withdrawn from the market, Corey M., who had been taking it for about eight months, began stockpiling it. The 30-year-old architect in Atlanta knew that Lotronex had caused serious side effects in some patients and had been linked to several deaths. But he had suffered no ill effects. On the contrary, Lotronex was the only drug that had ever helped him, stopping the severe pain and diarrhea caused by an illness called irritable bowel syndrome. "It was a miracle medicine for me," Corey said.[66]

Irritable bowel syndrome may not sound like a major disease, but it can cause substantial pain and interfere with normal living. "People are talking about serious life issues such as being able to keep a job and function on a daily basis, or just go out of the house," Jason Brodsky, a spokesman for the FDA, told the *Times*. "Their lives were changed by the medication."[67]

For thirty years I have been amazed that the drug industry and FDA have not fashioned a way of introducing new, potentially beneficial but risky drugs more safely—and, therefore, more successfully. The way the system has worked, once a drug is approved, just about anything goes. "Once a drug reaches the market," the *Times* reported, "aggressive promotion to doctors and advertising to consumers often lead to rapid growth in sales, so that, as in the case of Lotronex, hundreds of thousands of people are taking a new drug just months after its approval."[68]

This all-or-nothing system is risky to everyone—patients, physicians, drug companies, and the FDA. New drugs like Rezulin, Lotronex, Duract, and many others weren't needed by all of the patients who received them. Rezulin, with early evidence of liver injury, should not have been marketed toward all non-insulin-dependent diabetics. Instead, it should have been offered initially for people who absolutely needed a new approach—people for whom the benefits might well have been worth the risks. Lotronex could have been targeted toward severe cases or to patients unresponsive to other current therapies.

Instead, patients have died, while others, responding well to Lotronex or Rezulin, were denied vital treatment after the drugs were withdrawn. The manufacturers have lost valuable products. And the FDA is criticized from without and within.

"The pharmaceutical industry and the FDA need better sets of tools to handle safety issues that might come up once a drug is approved," said Dr. Victor Raczkowski, deputy director of the FDA office evaluating gastrointestinal drugs, including Lotronex. "This is relatively new territory for the industry and the FDA."[69]

But it shouldn't be new territory. As every chapter of this book has documented, improper dosages, unsafe drugs, and overly aggressive marketing have been causing avoidable side effects and unnecessary deaths for decades. Hasn't anyone at the FDA noticed before?

Belatedly, the FDA and Glaxo Wellcome began discussing methods of reintroducing Lotronex in a more supervised manner. The possibilities included limiting Lotronex to specific types of patients, or allowing only sanctioned specialists to prescribe it, or releasing it as an investigational drug with tight requirements for following patients. However, none of these will adequately protect patients unless a basic problem is addressed: Lotronex is one-size-fits-all. Patients young and old, big and small, healthy and ill—all receive the same Lotronex dosage. Patients with mild irritable bowel syndrome receive the same dosage as patients with severe disease. Certainly, Lotronex is one drug that should be started very low and increased gradually to ensure that no patient receives an iota more than she requires. Irritable bowel syndrome is rarely an emergency, so the "start low, go slow" approach makes sense and maximizes safety. But that's not how it is done in today's medical-pharmaceutical complex. So, inevitably, some people will be overmedicated if one-size-fits-all Lotronex enters the market again.

LIMITING INFORMATION is a strategy not only of the drug companies: Today's FDA also seems to have decided that limiting information is a way to limit criticism. When Raxar, a dangerous and unneeded antibiotic was finally withdrawn, the FDA minimized the media coverage by issuing no public statement whatsoever, a deviation from previous policy.[70] The FDA dampened the tide of criticism when it withdrew Regulen and Propulsid, a top-selling drug for seven years that was removed because of 80 deaths and 347 cardiac emergencies,[68] and when it withdrew Rezulin by making the announcements late in the day. This allowed the agency to avoid coverage on evening news programs and to limit the time for reporters to obtain independent experts' opinions for the next day's newspaper stories.[71]

The FDA is also limiting opposition on the front end—during the approval process. In January 1999, Public Citizen sued the FDA to obtain access to information presented at FDA advisory committee meetings.[72] Although the committee members were provided with studies and reports about the drugs they were considering, the public was denied timely access to this information. In a policy straight out of Kafka, the public was invited to make comments at these meetings, but before the information from drug-company studies and FDA analyses was released. Dr. Sidney Wolfe, the director of Public Citizen's Health

Research Group, stated: "Not only does this flawed policy of secrecy pay phony lip service to public participation in what is legally a public process, but it also has potentially serious negative consequences to the public health."[73]

Dr. Wolfe wasn't exaggerating. In June 2000, an FDA advisory committee held public hearings on applications for approval of low-dose, over-the-counter versions of Mevacor and Pravachol. I was interested in these applications because I expected that the studies supporting low-dose Mevacor and Pravachol would show that many people with mild cholesterol disorders did not require the higher doses that physicians typically prescribe (Chapter 6). However, I couldn't find any information about these applications. In essence, although the FDA invited public testimony, it did not provide any specific information about what the companies were requesting. How, then, could a person evaluate the merit of these applications? Ultimately this information was made public—the day of the hearings—too late for me to be scheduled or to provide informed input at the hearings.

Without adequate information on drugs being considered for approval, "public" hearings are shams.

IT IS EASY to see why morale at the FDA is low.[74] Having drugs approved against the recommendations of evaluating officers and seeing these drugs harm thousands of people have taken their toll. Many respected FDA officers have left the agency.

Even in better times, working for the FDA is a difficult job. FDA officers have to make difficult decisions about drugs, all of which are probably going to harm some fraction of the population. When an FDA doctor must decide whether to recommend approval of a new drug, relatively little is actually known about the drug, and nearly all of what is known is from the drug company's research. And while the FDA deliberates, the drug companies are pressuring and their congressional supporters are lobbying, and the consumer groups and the media are watching. The pharmaceutical industry donated $44 million to the major political parties in the last decade.[75] In 1992, Congress required the FDA to speed up the review process, and drug-approval times have been reduced 50 percent. In interviews with FDA medical personnel, the *Los Angeles Times* found: "The FDA reviewers said they and their bosses fear that unless drugs are approved, [the drug] companies will erupt and Congress will retaliate by refusing to renew user fees. This would cripple FDA operations—and jeopardize jobs."[76]

Of course, the FDA can always send a new drug back for more studies, but what about the people who are ill or dying while the new drug receives months or years of further analysis? Withholding a drug too long can be as harmful as approving it too quickly. Choosing between speed and safety isn't easy, and sometimes there is no happy medium. Meanwhile the FDA is often criticized for going too slow and for going too quickly. "The FDA is in a corner," said Dr. Lammer, director of medical genetics at the Children's Center of Northern California, in Oakland. "They either get nailed by the pharmaceutical industry for keeping a drug off market, or they let it on and it's a free-for-all."[77]

Now add an annual deficit that approaches $200 million, causing massive shortages in personnel and equipment, and the result is an agency in disarray. This disarray became public in August 2000 following an article by FDA Commissioner Jane Henney in *USA Today*. Dr. Henney's opinion piece was meant to reassure the public about FDA protections for people volunteering for new drug studies.[78] In previous months, evidence had surfaced that in many of these studies, volunteers had not received adequate supervision or been given proper informed consent. Because of these and other shortcomings, volunteers had died. But not everyone was buying Henney's assurances—not even at the FDA. Dr. Robert Misbin, who had been one of the first to come forward during the Rezulin debacle, immediately rebutted Henney's claims. In an open letter to *USA Today* three weeks later, Misbin pointed out that although Henney claimed the FDA would ensure the protection of study subjects, she offered no policies for carrying this out. Indeed, Misbin said, Henney missed an excellent opportunity to back up her words when "the FDA ignored a finding that written informed consent had not been properly obtained from approximately 300 patients who participated in trials of the new diabetes drug Avandia."[79]

Misbin added, "The FDA could have sent a message to the pharmaceutical industry that it took informed consent seriously. Missing this opportunity was not simply an oversight. To the contrary, I was advised not to bring up the informed-consent problem at a public meeting of the FDA advisory committee where the Avandia application was being discussed. Although Henney states that her obligation to protect patients' rights is 'deeply felt,' her method of implementing that obligation seems designed to be ineffective."[80]

A STATEMENT by Dr. Janet Woodcock and other officers of the FDA Center for Drug Evaluation and Research in November 2000 was encouraging:

> These experiences have catalyzed an evolution in our thinking on risk management and the evaluation of new drugs for approval. The FDA's risk assessment must evaluate both the drug's intrinsic safety profile as well as the ability of the health care system to adequately manage known toxicities.[81]

Proving that she had gotten the picture, Woodcock added, "The public has a strong desire for safe drugs."

However, subsequent steps by the FDA are not as encouraging. In December 2000 the FDA announced an initiative to improve package inserts so that the most important information is easier for physicians and patients to locate. This is a welcome step, but at the same time the FDA proposed limiting the list of adverse effects to only those "for which there is reasonable possibility that the product caused the response."[82] This clause is intended to sound reasonable enough, but in fact it would create a giant loophole by which drug companies and their hired researchers could explain away many important side effects and further minimize the risks of new drugs.

Not nearly enough is known about new drugs to offer reasonable explanations for every adverse reaction observed during early research. Physicians and patients have a right to know about each and every adverse effect experienced by study subjects during early research, no matter if the adverse effect was reasonably explainable or not at the time. Otherwise, important medication reactions will not be listed in new drugs' package inserts or *PDR* descriptions.

Physicians and patients depend on these listings to identify and handle problems that develop when millions of patients are suddenly taking new drugs after FDA approval. The present system allows drug companies to list side effects as infrequent or possibly not related to the drug itself. Isn't this enough to protect the interests of drug companies? What about the interests of patients?

In March 2001, I sent a letter to the FDA stating my opposition to allowing drug companies, with their major conflicts of interest, to explain away any medication side effect and thereby keep physicians and patients uninformed. By May, the FDA had not released its decision.

Needed Reforms in the FDA's Requirements for Drug Research, Development, and Marketing

1. Better dosage studies. Dosage studies must be thorough. The lowest effective doses must be clearly defined. The variation among patients would be fully delineated. Clear dosage and individual variation information must be required in the "Dosage and Administration" section of every package insert and *PDR* description, where doctors would most likely see it. Starting with a low dosage and individualizing the dosage must be emphasized, when medically appropriate.

2. Better methods for determining effectiveness. No more false comparisons with inadequate dosages of competitors' drugs or with older, less effective drugs. No more definitions of effectiveness that have little to do with the actual clinical uses of drugs or the needs of patients. The FDA would amend its methods of measuring effectiveness so that it did not lead drug companies to use higher dosages than actually needed by patients.

3. Better side-effect data. Methods of obtaining side-effect information would improve. The drug companies would have to show that its researchers specifically asked about all likely side effects with new drugs. Questionnaires would cover a wide range of less likely side effects, because many side effects cannot be anticipated, and because study subjects often do not relate unusual side effects unless specifically asked. Independent review would be required to exclude any side effects occurring during drug studies, rather than allowing drug-company–funded researchers to simply exclude those that they don't think were related to the drug.

4. Better research on the elderly, women, and adolescents. Thorough research regarding the responses of different groups such as adolescents, women, and the elderly should be required with any drug marketed for general usage.

5. Research should be conducted on likely patients. The effect of alcohol on Viagra was studied only in healthy people, but most men taking Viagra have other disorders, such as hypertension, cardiovascular disease, or obesity, and often they are taking other medications.

Studies of drug interactions and other important factors should be done on typical patients. The responses of women should also be evaluated and reported.

6. All important information should be included in the package insert and PDR. Presently, package inserts and *PDR* descriptions contain the information that the drug companies and the FDA agree upon. A great deal of important information is omitted. The drug companies should include all important data in their product information: all effective dosages, all side effects, all drug interactions, and potential drug interactions that weren't studied. Product information should be updated annually as new findings accrue after new drugs are approved.

7. Conflicts of interest should be curtailed and made public. Doctors performing vital studies or involved in making decisions about the approval of a new drug should not be permitted to have financial ties with the manufacturer. FDA advisory committees should exclude doctors with ties to the manufacturers of medications being reviewed. If the expert input of physicians with drug-company ties are necessary, the conflicts of interest must be made public.

8. Proprietary information—information kept from the public—should be limited. Drug companies should withhold information crucial to maintaining their patents and production methods, but all other data from animal and clinical studies should remain in the public domain. Drug companies should not be allowed to hide information just because it was unfavorable. Unfavorable findings are often crucial to recognizing dangers of new drugs and assuring the public's safety. All dosage and safety studies should be published or made available by request.

9. FDA powers over pharmaceutical advertising would be strengthened. Drug advertising must be balanced and accurate. The FDA should be able to levy stiff penalties on advertisers that mislead the public about medications.

What the FDA Shouldn't Do: Why We Need an Independent Medication Safety Monitoring System

THE REZULIN, LOTRONEX, SELDANE, Propulsid, Posicor, Duract, and other disasters reveal another serious obstacle to a truly effective FDA. The agency's officials must work not only under constant pressure, but also with unavoidable conflicts of interest. Even if every FDA official began with a neutral attitude regarding the drug companies, inherent conflicts of interest would soon develop.

An FDA doctor spends months or years evaluating a new drug. If he ultimately recommends approval, he is going to be professionally and emotionally invested in the performance of the new drug. Like an author finally publishing a book, an FDA medical officer wants a medication he shepherds through the approval process to perform well. Also, the FDA doctor has spent a great deal of time with drug-company representatives and researchers. At the very least, he has developed professional relationships with some of these people, and he knows how important the drug is to their company and careers.

If a drug fails, it is extremely disappointing as well as personally em-barrassing for the FDA official. He must answer, sometimes publicly, for recommending the approval of a drug that may have harmed or killed people. Human nature is such that this may be very difficult for him to accept. It is always possible to find some good with a drug, and this can provide a basis for maintaining that the drug should be kept on the market. Under these circumstances, the FDA is probably the last agency that should be judging newly discovered risks after a drug is marketed. Or, as Drs. Alastair Wood, Raymond Woosley, and C. M. Stein wrote in 1998 in *The New England Journal of Medicine,* the recom-mendation of FDA officials "for approval involves substantial personal identification with that approval, and it is unlikely that those who rec-ommended a drug for approval could later conduct a dispassionate evaluation of possible harm due to that drug."[1] Authors of a 1998 ar-ticle in *JAMA* agreed: "The discovery of serious adverse effects not de-tected in pre-approval testing can be unwelcome news to both the drug's sponsor and the FDA division that evaluated and approved the drug."[2]

I believe that this is precisely what happened with Rezulin, as we saw in Chapter 11. Drs. Woodcock, Lumpkin, and other top officials had placed themselves on the line in fast-tracking Rezulin. Admitting failure with the drug meant admitting the failure of their fast-track policy. It must have been very difficult—maybe impossible, based on their continuing denials regarding the seriousness of Rezulin's haz-ards and their rationalizations for the ineffective steps they took while delaying Rezulin's withdrawal for years.

Most worrisome is that some of them are still making excuses, in-sisting that the process worked properly. If so, why did it take the FDA more than two years longer than British authorities to act? To inter-vene to save dozens, perhaps hundreds, of lives? This is a recurring problem at the FDA.

WHAT SHOULD BE DONE? Drs. Wood, Woosley, and Stein an-swered this question in their 1998 article "Making Medicines Safer: The Need for An Independent Medication Safety Board."[3] They pointed out that in other vital areas of government oversight—investigating airline crashes, railroad accidents, and toxic spills—independent agencies exist to perform objective, in-depth investigations. Yet, although medication reactions cause more injuries, disabilities, and deaths than all of the airline, railroad, environmental, and automobile accidents combined, no independent agency exists to monitor and investigate them.

From 1995 to 1997, only 511 fatalities occurred on U.S. airlines, but each was investigated by the National Transportation Safety Board, and public hearings were held. However, deaths from drug reactions occur many times more frequently than from airplane accidents, but we do not have a system performing similar types of investigations involving medication reactions. Our current reporting system is entirely voluntary and inadequate. The monitoring conducted by the FDA is, as Wood et al. put it, "based on the assumption that a drug is safe unless case reports of adverse effects call that assumption into question."[4]

Case reports are a very shaky barometer by which to gauge the dangers of medications. Only about 5 percent of adverse reactions ever get reported to the FDA.[5,6] Some experts believe only 1 percent are reported.[7,8] "Most doctors don't know the system exists," Dr. Brian Strom, an expert in the department of biostatistics and epidemiology at the University of Pennsylvania, told *The New York Times* in 1997.[9] Hospitals are also supposed to report adverse drug events, but as Dr. David Bates wrote in *JAMA*, "Hospitals have had strong incentives not to identify too many of these events. Reporting large numbers of adverse events and any serious preventable event brings intense scrutiny from regulators and the public."[10] In addition, some drug reactions are very difficult to recognize. Seldane's cardiac toxicity, for example, was subtle and unrecognized for years, so many heart arrhythmias and deaths this drug caused were probably never identified or reported. Overall, the result is that the vast majority of medication reactions go unrecognized officially.

Even so, the FDA cannot handle the thousands of reports it does receive each week. There is not enough staff to tabulate these reports in a manner that would reveal anything less than an obvious problem. According to Dr. Curt Furberg, chairman of the department of public health sciences at the Bowman Gray School of Medicine, in 1997 the FDA had only fifty-five employees directly charged with postmarketing drug surveillance, and only a few of them had advanced degrees.[11] In March 2000, *The New York Times* asked Dr. Robert Fenichel, formerly an FDA officer for eleven years, about the adequacy of the FDA's postmarketing drug monitoring. He replied, "We have many, many more drugs than we used to that are out there, and the same budget is being used to follow them. It's being done less well."[12]

In contrast, the FAA and the Nuclear Regulatory Commission and similar agencies employ thousands of people. "It's all paid for by the industry that's monitored," Dr. Furberg said. "The only exception is prescription drugs."[13] The drug companies pay fees for the actual review of a new drug by the FDA, but the law "prohibits the agency from spending these fees on post-marketing surveillance or other drug-safety programs," as Wood, Stein, and Woosley wrote.[14] An article in *The New England Journal of Medicine* added: "Although the FDA collects spontaneous reports of suspected adverse effects . . . , except in unusual circumstances the FDA cannot fund, conduct, or require controlled postmarketing studies."[15]

THE LIMITATIONS OF the FDA monitoring system became obvious to me when, through the Freedom of Information Act, I ordered the FDA's adverse drug reports on several medications. I was sent information so disorganized that I would never accept such work from a graduate student. But with insufficient staff to process the quarter of a million reports involving three or four thousand drugs it receives each year, the FDA cannot perform proper ongoing analysis, and many reports are simply given numbers and filed away. A drug receives proper attention only when the number of problems becomes too big to miss or until some other party—a medical center, a newspaper, a consumer health group—points the way.

That's exactly what happened with Rezulin. The FDA didn't recognize the problem. The *Los Angeles Times* did, and even then the FDA was slow to react. Still, despite the fact that the FDA's ability to perform adequate postmarketing drug monitoring is greatly hindered by underfunding and understaffing, Congress has repeatedly refused to provide additional funding or to require the pharmaceutical industry to pay for monitoring its products.[16] This is why, in 1998, Dr. Thomas J. Moore wrote in *JAMA:* "The drug industry should be no less liable for the costs of its safety regulation than the nuclear industry, which pays for the full costs of the Nuclear Regulatory Commission . . . This investment in drug safety has potential to save thousands of lives and prevent tens of thousands of serious injuries every year."[17]

In comparison, France has thirty separate, fully staffed monitoring centers spread across a country smaller than Texas for the specific purpose of monitoring drug utilization and for responding quickly to problems. As Dr. Woosley wrote to me: "It's a question of priorities."

THE DIVISION OF government responsibilities for air travel safety provides a good model for how drug evaluation and monitoring systems could be organized. The Federal Aviation Administration (FAA) is responsible for air traffic control and other air travel activities. However, air crash investigations are conducted by the National Transportation Safety Board, an investigatory agency that is independent of the FAA. With this in mind, Wood et al. suggested that an independent National Medication Safety Board should be established to conduct ongoing analyses and to take swift action when problems with approved drugs arise.

What could a National Medication Safety Board accomplish? It wouldn't take much to improve on the current FDA system. Just going from crisis to crisis, trying to put out one brush fire after another, is sometimes more than the FDA can accomplish. That's why, after the FDA made its first comprehensive report on hundreds of deaths associated with Viagra in November 1998 and then required new warnings in the Viagra labeling, no subsequent FDA reports have been forthcoming. I was stunned when I learned that the FDA had suspended its analysis of Viagra, a drug linked with nearly 500 deaths in just thirteen months. I shouldn't have been, because Drs. Tom Moore, Bruce Psaty, and Curt Furberg had written in *JAMA:*

Neither the FDA nor any other agency has an organized program to find out whether the important warning messages are
achieving their intended purpose of protecting the public and,
if not, discovering the cause. . . . Instead of waiting passively for
spontaneous reports, active surveillance involves looking for
sensitive indicators of possible problems.[18]

They also reminded readers that inadequate FDA monitoring had
been a problem for more than thirty years.

The need for independent safety monitoring has been long recognized. In 1970, a National Academy of Sciences panel recommended establishing a National Drug Surveillance Center
reporting directly to the FDA commissioner. In 1980 the Joint
Commission on Prescription Drug Use recommended to Congress the creation of a Center for Drug Surveillance completely
separate from the FDA.[19]

So, in 1998, although Pfizer and the FDA acted as if all concerns
about Viagra had been settled, I wasn't convinced. That's why I did
the analysis comparing Viagra to Caverject (Chapter 4), another drug
for treating erectile dysfunction. I found that Viagra was linked to
more than five times as many reports of deaths to the FDA as Caverject. This was a very significant difference. The fact that a solitary, un-
funded doctor like me had to perform such an obvious analysis—that
the FDA hadn't considered such a simple comparison for a drug that
has been linked to so many deaths—is ridiculous.

A National Medication Safety Board (NMSB) could monitor approved drugs on an ongoing basis and identify problems quickly, preventing them from becoming major crises. When a crisis does arise,
the NMSB could perform in-depth analyses and hold public hearings,
just as the National Transportation Safety Board does following airplane crashes.

The NMSB could also enact new measures to maximize prevention. It could ensure that doctors and patients receive full information regarding drug doses, side effects, and safety measures. It could

ensure that the drug companies keep their product information current and complete, and that newly identified side effects are quickly added to the list. If necessary, it could facilitate new safety studies broader than the drug companies had done.

The NMSB could also facilitate comparative studies of drug safety among medications used for the same disease. It could undertake long-term monitoring for widely used drugs with brief track records. For example, millions of people will take Zocor, Lipitor, and other cholesterol-lowering drugs for decades, but our knowledge of these drugs' long-term effects and potential side effects is limited. The NMSB could keep a watchful eye on these and similar experiments that are now taking place in the general population. Government agencies evaluate airlines in terms of meeting arrival times, proper baggage handling, and overall safety; isn't the monitoring of drug safety at least as important?

The NMSB could also monitor advertising directed at physicians and consumers. It could ensure that the advertising was presented in an accurate and balanced manner. In addition, the NMSB could evaluate whether the impact of this advertising was beneficial in educating the public about available therapies for untreated conditions, or whether advertising spurred inappropriate medication use and unnecessary adverse effects. Presently the FDA has less than a dozen full-time staff to monitor advertising that amounts to approximately $14 billion a year in the United States.[20]

A NATIONAL MEDICATION Safety Board could also monitor what doctors are prescribing and at what doses by analyzing clusters of prescriptions, assuring confidentiality just as the FDA does with adverse reaction cases. Such monitoring would reveal whether doctors switch to lower, safer doses after studies are published that demonstrate their effectiveness. Or whether doctors know, for example, that the current standard of hypertension therapy is to start with lower doses than the drug companies recommend. Many doctors do not. Indeed, because of the poor dissemination of new information and because of inadequate medical school training in the intricacies of optimizing medication therapy, many physicians do not prescribe drugs properly or as safely as possible. Yet, no one is held responsible.

In 1995, Dr. Jerry Avorn, of the Harvard School of Public Health, wrote: "Once the FDA makes these drugs legally available, the agency emphatically rejects responsibility for overseeing how wisely or ineptly physicians prescribe them. . . . At present, literally no one has the responsibility for ensuring that physicians are indeed using drugs optimally."[21]

A National Medication Safety Board could monitor these issues and develop ways of informing doctors about important changes in the standards of care. Studies have shown that methods of prescribing medications and decisions about performing surgery vary widely from doctor to doctor and from state to state. These variations indicate outdated or inappropriate methods by many physicians. An NMSB could identify these problems and work to rectify them. Similarly, it could monitor doctors' medication selections and dosages and inform them of new studies offering better selections and lower doses.

A startling example of inadequate drug monitoring occurred with Coumadin (warfarin), a vital drug for the 750,000 Americans taking it annually. But using Coumadin is tricky because it thins the blood, and if the dosing is even slightly high, hemorrhaging can occur. Therefore, Coumadin is reserved for serious, potentially life-threatening disorders, and doctors monitor patients closely. Blood tests are taken regularly to gauge Coumadin's anticoagulation effect and to determine the proper dosage. But in the late 1960's and early 1970's, U.S. hospitals changed their tests for measuring the effects of Coumadin, which altered the test results—which in turn sometimes caused physicians to prescribe the wrong doses of Coumadin. Even at proper doses, the risks with Coumadin are considerable, and people can bleed out "from any tissue or organ," as DuPont Pharma describes it. Improper dosing increases the risks.

In 1987 the *Archives of Internal Medicine* published "Is the Dose of Warfarin Prescribed by American Physicians Unnecessarily High?"[22] In it, Dr. Jack Hirsh warned doctors that the skewed Coumadin tests were causing the undertreatment or overtreatment of thousands of people, exposing them either to recurrences of their disorders or to the serious risks of Coumadin overmedication. More often it was the latter. Moreover, not only did people using different laboratories get different test results, but even those using the same lab for their tests sometimes got completely different results—and therefore completely different Coumadin doses—even though the amount they actually needed hadn't changed at all.

Dr. Hirsh wrote: "For more than two decades many patients in North America could have been treated as effectively but more safely by using lower doses of oral anticoagulants." How much more safely? For just one of Coumadin's uses, treating venous thromboembolism, each year 43,000 cases of "clinically important bleeding" were occurring that could have been prevented.[23] These reactions included rectal bleeding, blood in the urine, bleeding beneath the skin and collecting into knots, profuse vaginal bleeding, and severe bleeding from the nose. Some patients had to be hospitalized. If all patients taking Coumadin for various conditions were included, about 130,000 avoidable, significant hemorrhages from excessive doses of Coumadin were occurring annually. Over fifteen to twenty years, that's more than two million avoidable, serious drug reactions.

Unfortunately, little changed after Hirsh's article. In fact, this wasn't Hirsh's first warning to the medical community. In 1982 he and others had published a similar warning in *The New England Journal of Medicine*.[24] Yet, even after publication in this highly respected publication, little changed.

By 1990, Coumadin's manufacturer, DuPont, had incorporated many of the recommendations of Hirsh and other experts into the Coumadin package insert and the *PDR*, advising doctors about the problems with the current methods of measuring Coumadin anticoagulation. DuPont also recommended lower Coumadin doses. Still, by 1993, so little had changed that *The New England Journal of Medicine* published another warning by Eckman et al.: "The more than half a million Americans receiving long-term anticoagulant therapy face unnecessary risks of bleeding or thromboembolism. . . ."[25] The article stated that about 1 percent of Coumadin-related hemorrhages caused permanent neurological damage, such as strokes. And how many deaths? The study didn't say, but likely hundreds each year. The article concluded: "With older recommendations, anticoagulation can actually have poorer prognoses than those who didn't receive it."[26] In other words, many people receiving Coumadin were in greater danger than people with the same conditions who refused treatment altogether.

Finally, by the mid-1990's, things began to improve. Laboratories began modernizing their Coumadin tests and standardizing their results according to an international scale adopted in Europe two decades earlier. In the summer of 1994, I asked the director of a hospital laboratory about the Coumadin epidemic. He said, "I didn't think it was a big deal when I first heard of it. I didn't realize the impact. After reading the articles dating back to '82, I thought, Geez, this is obvious. Why didn't people fix the problem?" He shook his head and added, "I'm lecturing at a big Los Angeles hospital next week. It's going to be a shock to the doctors. They are going to be amazed when they update their methods, how it's going to reduce the doses of Coumadin they prescribe."

An NMSB could have alerted physicians much faster than the twenty-five years it took for the system to adapt. It could have required adoption of the accurate standard applied in Europe decades earlier. It could have ensured that every physician was informed about the problem. This could have been accomplished with the assistance of medical organizations, hospitals, pharmacies, and laboratories—wherever Coumadin prescriptions were written or filled, and whenever the blood tests were conducted. As discussed in previous chapters, a huge information gap exists in the medical world. Information is rarely disseminated rapidly. It takes up to seventeen years for accepted changes in treatment to be adopted by the vast majority of physicians. With Coumadin, one of the riskiest drugs in use, it took even longer. An NMSB could bring organization to, and improve information dissemination in, this fragmented system.

WHEN YOU THINK about it, a National Medication Safety Board makes so much sense, it is hard to believe that no objective, independent governmental agency is consistently and reliably performing drug monitoring, enacting preventive procedures, ensuring the optimal treatment of patients, or undertaking any of the other functions listed at the end of this chapter. Yet, Phase 4, the postapproval phase of drug research when new drugs are released for general usage, is the most important and dangerous phase of all. Phase 4 is when we really learn the truth about new drugs. According to Dr. Moore, "Discovery of new dangers of drugs after marketing is common. Overall, 51% of approved drugs have serious adverse effects not detected prior to approval."[27]

Drug companies and the FDA know this. They know that we will learn a great deal about a new drug after it is prescribed to you and several million others. That's when a new drug's safety and effectiveness are really proven—or disproven. There's just no way to know these things from studies before FDA approval that involved just a few hundred or a few thousand subjects. Phase 4 involves millions of patients—but no one is actively monitoring it. Is it any wonder that people aren't better protected? Or that every week, new headlines announce another problem with our medications?

This is why Drs. Moore, Psaty, and Furberg concluded:

At a time when Congress recently passed legislation intended to make new drugs available more rapidly . . . a more active and effective safety program for marketed drugs is essential to protect the public health. . . . The nation needs an office of drug safety with the authority, independence, funds, and legal mandate to undertake all of the major tasks that define a basic drug safety monitoring program.[28]

Drs. Wood, Stein, and Woosley concurred:

We believe that a post-marketing drug-safety program that is independent of the agency responsible for drug approval (in the United States, the Food and Drug Administration) needs to be established. . . . Such independence is to ensure objectivity and to avoid conflicts of interest.[29]

There is one last urgent reason for creating a National Medication Safety Board. For many decades, the lengthy FDA procedure for approving new medications protected Americans in an unrecognized way. The best-remembered incident was the thalidomide disaster that led to severe birth defects in children. The United States was spared the full force of this tragedy because the drug's introduction here came long after thalidomide was approved in Europe. Thus, the first revelations and warnings came from Europe, where thalidomide did much more damage.

Now that the FDA, pressured by Congress, is fast-tracking new drugs and approving them with less research, Americans are often the first population in the world to be exposed. We can no longer look to Europe and other parts of the world as our early-warning systems. Instead, it is our own Phase 4 experience—performed on millions of people every day—that will warn the rest of the world. Drs. Wood, Stein, and Woosley sounded the alarm in 1998:

> The United States is now often the first country to approve new drugs, but neither the FDA nor the medical community has the infrastructure to detect, investigate, or prevent their unwanted consequences. The FDA clearly does not have the resources to identify problems associated with drugs, much less to determine the magnitude of the problems. . . .[30]

Now you know why it was the *Los Angeles Times,* not the FDA, that uncovered the Rezulin disaster.[31] And why it was I, not the FDA, who discovered that Viagra was linked to significantly more reported deaths than a comparative drug.[32] And that it was a persistent laboratory technician who, against initial skepticism of hospital physicians, sounded the alert about heart valve irregularities and serious, sometimes lethal pulmonary reactions with Fen-Phen and Redux. Now you know why the side-effect epidemic not only has persisted for decades, but isn't even acknowledged.

How a National Medication Safety Board Could Improve Medication Safety

A National Medication Safety Board (NMSB) could perform many activities to improve medication use and safety:

New Drug Monitoring

1. Begin monitoring new drugs as soon as they are approved in order to confirm that they are safe and effective.

2. Review all safety information from drug manufacturers and from independent studies as they appear in the medical literature.

3. Develop a reciprocal mechanism for sharing information with the National Institutes of Health and other research centers. These agencies would immediately notify the NMSB of any newly discovered drug toxicities during their studies.

4. Develop a centralized database that incorporates new drug safety information. This current and comprehensive information would be accessible to the health community and to the public.

Crisis Management

1. Provide ongoing scrutiny of drug reaction reports, using computer analyses to identify trends quickly.

2. Hold public hearings with representatives of the FDA, drug companies, physician groups, consumer health groups, and drug-safety specialists when public safety issues arise.

3. Issue regular, official reports regarding its findings.

4. Recommend actions necessary to maximize drug safety. This would include the power to place restrictions on how some drugs are used. For example, while Rezulin remained available, it should have been restricted to patients unresponsive to other, safer diabetes drugs. The NMSB could quickly remove drugs when necessary.

Develop and Enact Preventive Strategies

1. Develop measures for improving how doctors prescribe medications to patients.

2. Ensure that doctors receive all significant preapproval and postapproval information regarding the effective range of dosages for all drugs. Encourage doctors to adopt a flexible, individualized, patient-based approach when selecting doses.

3. Ensure that doctors and patients receive current and complete information about beneficial new effects and newly identified adverse effects with all approved drugs.

4. Ensure that drug companies make annual, comprehensive updates of their package inserts and *PDR* write-ups. This would ensure a complete, current, and accurate source of drug information.

Chapter 13

Doctors, Drugs, and Patients

I RECEIVE MANY e-mails and letters from patients asking about side effects that their doctors fail to acknowledge. Here's a typical one:

Could you tell me if you are getting a lot of people writing to you about Lipitor problems? I had lots of memory/mind problems, couldn't sleep, forgot what I was doing (including names, telephone numbers) and, later, muscle and joint pain on the 10 mg dose. My doctor refuses to believe that it could be the Lipitor even though the problems went away when I took myself off the stuff. I printed out some of the descriptions I found on the Web and showed my doctor, but again she said there were no studies showing these side effects and that these personal reports meant nothing.

Why did this doctor ignore the man's complaints? Why did she dismiss the information the man collected from the Internet? Why would this doctor, like so many doctors, accept the side-effect information from drug companies but so hastily dismiss the first-hand reports of her own patient?

Such cases are not limited to Lipitor patients. After a woman named Helen was prescribed Prozac, her sexual drive and ability to attain orgasm disappeared. The doctor said that Prozac wasn't the cause. She endured this for three years until reading a magazine article that informed her otherwise. Eli Lilly and Company's information on Prozac lists these side effects as infrequent, but attentive doctors know that Prozac causes sexual dysfunctions in about 50 percent of patients.

An elderly relative of mine was taking Prilosec for heartburn. Over the years, the arthritis in his hands became very painful. I mentioned that Prilosec can sometimes cause joint pains. He stopped the Prilosec and the pain disappeared. He had told his doctor about his increasing arthritis pain, but the doctor never connected the problem to the drug.

Each of these side effects was dose-related, stemming from standard drug-company doses. Each of these side effects was listed in the drugs' package inserts and *PDR* descriptions. They should have been easily recognizable and correctable, but instead they were missed or dismissed. One woman captured the feelings of many patients after her doctor ignored an important, obvious reaction to an antibiotic. "Doctors don't ask about side effects and don't want to hear about them. They would rather assume the problem is from some other cause, not the drug."

Although many physicians pay attention to side effects, many apparently do not, for I frequently receive complaints from patients about side effects that were readily identifiable. Yet, again and again, they were not identified or treated. Why?

When people refuse to see the obvious, it is called "denial." When a substantial segment of a profession repeatedly employs denial, something larger is going on. It is this: Many doctors overidentify with their medications. Perhaps, to some degree, this is natural. After all, the most common action that doctors take is to prescribe a medication. In 1999, doctors wrote 2.8 billion prescriptions—8 million prescriptions every day of the year. The ego-attachment of some doctors to their medications goes beyond reasonable, however, and becomes pernicious when they become defensive and dismissive about obvious, common side effects; when they uncritically accept biased information from the drug companies, then stonewall unbiased patients' legitimate complaints; and when their denial inadvertently allows drug companies to continue to market drugs that are inadequately researched, improperly produced, and dosed in ways that cause millions of avoidable side effects.

Doctors' intransigence harms more than individual patients. It harms the credibility of the profession and erodes its most important pillar—trust. The enormity of dissatisfaction and fear among patients is apparent in almost every aspect of medical care. One third of patients receiving prescriptions never fill them—hardly a testimonial of their comfort with their doctors' decisions. Fifty percent of people receiving medications for many serious conditions quit treatment, risking their long-term health and longevity as well as adding huge long-term costs to the health-care system. Millions more express greater confidence in unproven, unregulated health-store supplements that often do not contain the amounts listed on the labels than in standardized, regulated medications. These are sure signs that patients' concerns about medication are not being addressed.

A BIG PART of the problem is that doctors are inadequately trained about medications. Medical schools provide insufficient education about drugs or about the art of treating patients individually. Medical students are not taught how to critically evaluate drug studies, or about the deficiencies in drug-company information, or that standard drug-company doses are unnecessarily high for millions of patients. Thus, in 1995, Dr. Jerry Avorn, of the school of public health at Harvard, wrote:

There is an informational void about pharmaceuticals in the training of most doctors, despite the importance of the prescription in medical care. . . . Most of those who have looked

thoughtfully at this process have been appalled at its inadequacy. Despite the explosion of new and powerful agents available for use over the last two decades, during this same period
the teaching of clinical pharmacology and therapeutics has
been a waning endeavor at many American medical schools.[1]

Such criticisms are not new:

- *Journal of Clinical Pharmacology,* 1990: "The physician in clinical
  practice needs guidance. Decisions are being made based on anecdotal experiences or on sales promotion."[2]
- *Emergency Medicine and Acute Care Essays,* 1993: "The most casual
  review of the medical literature quickly makes it clear that physician prescribing practices leave much to be desired."[3]
- *The New England Journal of Medicine,* 1998: "Much of the morbidity
  and mortality currently associated with drug therapy is due to
  well-recognized adverse effects and reflects our inability as health
  professionals to implement current knowledge fully."[4]
- *JAMA,* 2000: "In this age of rapid communication and advanced
  medical care, how can contraindicated prescribing continue?
  How can caring physicians continue to prescribe drugs in ways
  that have been identified as dangerous and potentially harmful?"[5]

The result is that many physicians are not taught about the importance of fitting drug doses to the individual needs of patients. And
when dose-related side effects inevitably occur, doctors are not properly prepared to deal with patients' complaints or to simply lower the
doses. Instead, many doctors adopt an attitude of skepticism about
anything that doesn't conform to their information, most of which
comes from the drug companies.

"One of the hardest things to comprehend through all of this is the
ignorance of most doctors concerning these side effects," a 51-year-
old woman wrote to me. Previously healthy and athletic, she developed an infection after abdominal surgery. Levaquin, an antibiotic,
was prescribed, and within two days she began experiencing electrical
sensations and numbness in her legs. These symptoms were not im-

mediately recognized as side effects, so she was told to finish the twenty-one-day prescription. By that time, she had tendinitis in her shoulder and knee, a partially torn Achilles tendon, and impaired concentration and memory. She needed crutches for three months, and after a year the tendon and memory problems persisted. Although adverse reactions involving nerves, joints, and tendons are well documented with this antibiotic,[6] her physicians still dismissed the possibility of a drug reaction.

I received more than sixty similar reports from patients with severe reactions to fluoroquinolone antibiotics such as Levaquin, Cipro, and Floxin. Robert T. was a 42-year-old, previously active man when he received Levaquin for a prostate infection. Within three days he developed side effects, so he discontinued the drug. His doctor then prescribed Cipro—a bad choice because the two antibiotics are chemically related. The first dose of Cipro reignited the side effects, leaving Robert with intense muscle pain lasting five months, and neck pain and nerve problems lasting a year. These side effects have been reported with Cipro,[7,8] but none of Robert's doctors recognized this. "No doctor I spoke to found an organic problem or was sympathetic to the idea that I might be having an adverse reaction to these antibiotics," he told me.

SOMETIMES EVEN OBVIOUS solutions elude physicians who are overly reliant on drug-company methods. A friend's daughter was depressed. The doctor prescribed Paxil at the standard dose, 20 mg/day. This wasn't enough, so the doctor raised it to 30 mg/day, which resolved the depression but sedated the girl. Back and forth they went between 20 mg and 30 mg. Not once did it occur to the doctor to do the obvious: try 25 mg. This is basic common sense; even so, very few doctors ever think of such simple solutions. Why? Because doctors are trained to follow drug company recommendations, and with Paxil, the recommended doses are 10, 20, 30, and 40 mg. This dosage protocol is actually more gradual than the protocols of many other drugs, but a jump from 20 to 30 mg—a 50 percent increase—is still too much for some people. Yet, many doctors don't think about it in this fundamental way.

Perhaps the most insidious damage caused by doctors' overdependency on drug-company information is that they can become very close-minded about other possibilities. Many doctors aren't even willing to hear about better, safer dosages, even if these dosages have been proven medically and make sense logically. Thus, doctors unwittingly align themselves with the drug companies, becoming the purveyors and defenders of drug-company methods. If Pfizer recommends 10 mg of Lipitor initially for all users, or Searle recommends Celebrex 100 mg twice daily for everyone with osteoarthritis, or Schering produces Claritin at 10 mg for everyone age six and over (except for people with liver or kidney problems), then doctors assume that these irrational, one-size-fits-all guidelines must be correct. If drug companies do not recommend lower dosages, then these dosages must not be worth trying even with old or small patients, or with people with long histories of medication sensitivities.

If patients report side effects at drug-company dosages, so the thinking too often goes, obviously the drugs cannot be the culprits. The People's Pharmacy column, by Joe and Theresa Graedon, carried this report in December 2000: "My husband has been taking Zoloft and has experienced agitation, increased cholesterol levels, weight gain and manic behavior. His doctor says side effects are rare with this drug and doesn't want to prescribe anything else."[9] Agitation and weight gain are common side effects of Zoloft, the number-seven top-selling drug in America in 1999. Manic behavior can also occur and may become serious. For a doctor to miss such obvious, alarming side effects reveals either a shocking dearth of knowledge or an intransigence in admitting even basic problems with a medication.

Fortunately, not all doctors are close-minded. Following my December 6, 1999, article in *Newsweek* ("The One-Size Dose Does Not Fit All"),[10] I received several supportive letters from physicians. One doctor wrote, "As a physician who is a patient with chronic illness, I can tell you from my vast experience that the doses in the *PDR* are often way off. Further, taking more than one medication complicates dosing immeasurably."

The patients of one specialist kept telling her that the over-the-counter dose of Motrin (200 mg) worked fine for their rheumatoid arthritis. The doctor didn't know that studies in the 1960's and 1970's had repeatedly demonstrated the effectiveness of this low dose, because McNeil Pharmaceuticals did not market low-dose Motrin when the drug was approved by the FDA in 1974, and McNeil did not mention low-dose Motrin in its product information. Fortunately, the doctor listened to her patients.

"Patients tell me it works for them," this doctor told me. "They've convinced me. Other doctors think I'm practicing homeopathy."

This respected doctor was convinced by careful assessment of her patients' responses to low-dose medication, but she still couldn't convince other doctors. Something is very wrong when doctors' first response to a new idea that reduces patients' risks and costs is skepticism and disdain.

I encounter this same stance all of the time. So do other doctors concerned about these issues. A professor at the University of Southern California told me, "I am most distressed at the current practice of ritualized drug dosing. I have been interested in the importance of individualizing drug dosages since 1966, but I feel as though I am talking to the wind—no one cares to listen."

DOCTORS ALSO DISPLAY denial when, without any qualms, they prescribe drugs for long-term usage even though the drugs' long-term safety has not been assured. Of course, we cannot always wait years or decades for such assurances. Many people need treatment now. Yet, at the very least, doctors should tell the millions of patients who are taking Lipitor, Celebrex, Prilosec, Zoloft, and many other drugs that the long-term safety of these drugs has not been proven and that new side effects are often discovered years and decades after drugs are approved. People are entitled to informed consent, and providing it is a basic tenet of medical ethics.

However, many doctors omit this step. As we have seen, some doctors just don't want to deal with the unpleasant aspects of medication therapy, so they minimize or ignore them. The problem is that by disregarding the lack of long-term information, doctors also ignore the importance of using the very lowest effective long-term doses. Instead, patients are placed at unnecessary risks. Are these risks real? Consider just a few of the reports in medical journals:

- *Lancet,* Dec. 1999: After forty years of experience, the antibiotic erythromycin has now been linked to serious abdominal obstructions in infants.[11]
- *British Medical Journal,* Oct. 1999: Antidepressants such as Prozac, Paxil, Zoloft, trazodone, and others have now been linked to increased bleeding. Most cases are mild, but "it may be more serious, involving gastrointestinal, genitourinary, or intracranial bleeding."[12] Concomitant use of anti-inflammatory drugs including aspirin increases the risk even more.
- *American Journal of Epidemiology,* May 2000: After being used for five decades, a study suggests that tricyclic antidepressants (e.g., imipramine, amitriptyline) may be associated with increased rates of breast cancer. So may be Paxil, a new SSRI antidepressant.[13]
- *Journal of Clinical Psychopharmacology,* June 2000: The top-selling drug Clozapine has now been linked to sudden death in patients.[14]
- *Primary Psychiatry,* Sept. 2000: After nearly five decades of usage, Mellaril has been linked to cardiac arrhythmias. This problem was identified thirty years ago but only recently rediscovered by accident. Now, finally, Novartis warns that Mellaril should be used only when safer drugs are ineffective.[15]

Long-term side effects are not only a possibility, but a probability. This statement from *JAMA,* quoted in Chapter 1, bears repeating: "Discovery of new dangers of drugs after marketing is common. Overall, 51 percent of approved drugs have serious adverse effects not detected prior to approval."[16] The risks can be reduced by providing fully informed consent and using the very lowest effective doses. Unfortunately, many doctors do not provide either.

Dr. Sidney Wolfe, in writing about the causes of so many side effects in seniors, summed up the situation: "The lack of adequate testing and label information from the companies combined with the grossly inadequate amount of training that doctors get about prescribing for older adults result in dangerous misprescribing and overprescribing."[17] He is right—and regarding not only seniors, but all patients.

DOCTORS CAN BE particularly indifferent toward so-called "minor" side effects. "Minor" side effects—insomnia, headaches, dizziness, stomach pain, constipation, depression, joint pains, weakness, abnormal tastes, blurred vision, impotence, dry mouth, flatulence, sweating, sedation, etc.—cause major discomfort or distress for millions of people. Minor side effects can make normal functioning difficult and greatly reduce people's quality of life. And far more than major side effects, they drive people from treatment.

Still, if drug companies label these side effects as minor, that's what many doctors believe and tell patients. Patients take these side effects seriously and resent doctors' casual attitudes. Every day, it seems, I'm told another story of doctors denying or dismissing side effects that really vex people. To these people, when doctors irrationally deny or dismiss their honest complaints, the message is clear: Doctors' first allegiance is not to their patients, but to the medications they prescribe.

This allegiance explains why, rather than openly and objectively discussing the benefits and risks of medications, doctors gild the lily, emphasizing the benefits and minimizing or not even mentioning the risks. "Traditionally, doctors have told their patients little about possible unwanted effects of prescribed medicines," a 1992 study in the *British Medical Journal* found. "Only a quarter of patients knew what side effects their medicines could cause, and half of these 'informed' patients became aware of problems only when they themselves were affected."[18]

In December 1999 a group led by Dr. Clarence Braddock, of the departments of medicine and health services at the University of Washington, published in *JAMA* their results from videotaping physicians during office visits. Their findings revealed that primary-care doctors adequately discussed the benefits and risks of medical treatment with only 9 percent of their patients. The authors concluded that most patients did not receive enough information to fulfill their rights for informed consent.[19]

Yet, if a doctor withholds vital information about a drug's risks that causes harm, patients often have little recourse. Hard to believe, but in many states, doctors are not legally required to inform patients about side effects. When I learned about this, I contacted the medical board in California. True enough, physicians are not legally required to inform patients about the side effects of drugs. Instead, the responsibility is given to pharmacists. But although pharmacists are capable of reciting a list of standard side effects, they know little about the people purchasing the drugs. They know little about these patients' medical histories or individual medication tolerances. This cleaving of responsibility is unsound and guarantees problems. It is the physician who knows the patient and who is prescribing the medication—it should be the physician who discusses side effects.

DOCTORS' MOUNTING CONFLICTS of interest are revealed most readily today by repeated failures to provide informed consent to patients participating in drug-company–sponsored research at medical institutions. The media has reported on many research studies in which patients were not properly informed about the risks or about doctors' financial ties to the sponsoring companies or to the products being studied. The problem has become so widespread that in January 2001, the U.S. Department of Health and Human Services, led by former HHS Secretary Donna Shalala, proposed a working draft of new guidelines for drug-company–sponsored research at medical schools, hospitals, and research institutes. Yet, as reported by *Science Magazine,* Shalala's proposal, although merely a starting point for discussion, was roundly criticized by academic institutions.[20]

In February 2001, a committee consisting of leaders from major universities across the country released their own set of guidelines for institutions conducting drug-company research. Harvard Medical School dean Joseph B. Martin stated, "While academic-industry collaborations are essential if patients are to benefit from the current biomedical revolution, the integrity of those relationships must be monitored by policies that are clearer and more stringent than the norm today."[21] These guidelines received a better initial reception, but by mid-2001 their fate remained unclear. Nor was it clear how much impact, if any, these voluntary guidelines would have on ensuring that patients in research studies receive proper informed consent and monitoring.

WHO BENEFITS THE most from doctors' deficient knowledge about medications and defensive posture regarding side effects? The drug companies. If doctors tell patients about a drug's benefits while omitting or minimizing the risks—well, this amounts to excellent salesmanship. If doctors turn a deaf ear to side effects—well, this protects the marketability of side-effect–prone drugs. Finally, if doctors accept drug-company dosages as the best and only choices, and if they accept incomplete side-effect listings as accurate, they will defend medications they prescribe when problems arise—a great way to protect inadequate or biased drug-company research.

Most doctors don't think of themselves as allying with drug companies or protecting the pharmaceutical industry's interests, but this is the result. Doctors' uncritical acceptance of drug-company information, side-effect data, and unnecessarily high dosages not only feed the side-effect epidemic, but also allow drug companies to keep operating in exactly the same harmful manner.

"The feeling I get," Dr. Tony Weisenberger, a medication expert and a former medical director of a hospital in North Carolina, told me, "is that most doctors say to themselves, 'A 30-percent side-effect rate isn't too bad,' and they just accept it that 30 percent—and sometimes far more—of their patients are going to run into trouble. They just take it as a part of the job."

In other words, they accept and adopt the drug-industry line that side effects are inevitable and there's not much that can be done about them. Provoking side effects in 30 to 50 percent of patients becomes not only acceptable, but a reasonable standard of care. This is why your doctor may not be very moved by your side effects.

Of course, if physicians aren't informed about side effects because the data are suppressed during early research and side effects discovered later are not listed in drug references, it makes physicians' jobs more difficult. Thus, the *Hazards of Medications* states, "Concern for the patient is not enough. The physician must also have the necessary education, facilities and information to enable him to avoid adverse drug reactions and interactions."[22] And the information to identify medication reactions when they occur.

MY SENSE IS that many doctors are unaware of the extent that drug companies influence them. With less time than ever to handle their daily caseloads, doctors often don't have the luxury of reading a lot of journals or researching in the huge Medline database. Doctors rely on information that is readily available to them. The drug companies know this and make sure that they are the main source of this information. But sometimes, doctors are lax even about using information that is readily accessible.

Sheila works for a drug company. Her son, who has a congenital heart defect, developed swelling after starting a new drug. Sheila called the doctor, who insisted that "the drug could not cause the edema and that it was more likely attributable to heart failure." Sheila took the boy to the hospital, where no heart failure was found, but the doctors insisted the reaction wasn't drug-related. Sheila demanded that the resident physician obtain the package insert and, sure enough, edema in the extremities was a side effect in about 1 percent of patients taking the drug.

"So, here I was," she told me, "afraid my son was dying all for lack of a physician knowing what the drug does. I feel that physicians should make themselves more aware, but I have also observed drug salesmen in action and know that physicians have an expectation that salespeople have integrity. They tout the 'benefits' not as potential, but as if the benefits are an absolute given, and they never mention the adverse reactions."

Physicians have their own problems today. As Dr. James Dalen, editor in chief of the *Archives of Internal Medicine*, wrote in 2000:

Physicians are caught in the middle . . . Physicians have lost the ability to guide the care of their patients. Nearly every major medical decision that they make must be approved by the managed care plan, prospectively or retrospectively. In addition, physicians face an incredible "hassle factor." The managed care plan monitors their decisions—if they are found to be "outliers" with regard to their practice patterns [e.g., not seeing patients quickly enough], they face financial penalties or disenrollment.[23]

Patients are sympathetic to these pressures on physicians, but these problems are no excuse for failing to employ fundamental medical principles in treating patients. They do not excuse adopting a defensive, dismissive mindset toward patients' complaints or failing to even check whether a medication side effect is listed in available references.

Dr. David Kessler, the former commissioner of the FDA and presently the dean of the Yale University School of Medicine, was asked about the inadequacy in identifying medication reactions in the U.S. He replied, "The real issue, probably more important than the system, is for people to be looking, to be on guard, to be looking for possible associations of drugs with reactions."[24]

Being on guard means having an open mind. It means understanding that any medication can cause any reaction in any patient. The lists of side effects in package inserts and the *PDR* are not complete. Many side effects are not recognized in early research. Unfavorable findings in drug-company studies are sometimes suppressed. Many side effects recognized after FDA approval and widespread use are never incorporated into the *PDR*. This is why the *American Medical Association Drug Evaluations* advised physicians: "When prescribing newly released drugs, particular attention must be given to dosage and adverse effects."[25] This means any and all possible side effects.

Studies have repeatedly shown that when physicians are assiduous in monitoring for adverse effects in their patients, they identify far more side effects than otherwise. Identifying side effects isn't difficult. Guidelines exist. If an otherwise stable patient suddenly develops symptoms in close association with the use of a medication, and there are no other factors to explain the symptoms, and the symptoms abate when the drug is discontinued, this is a "probable" adverse drug effect.[26] The medication should be considered the likely cause—even if it isn't listed in the *PDR* or any other drug reference.

"All science is rooted in observations," wrote Dr. Robert Brodell, of the Case Western Reserve University School of Medicine, in August 2000, "and full-time physicians are in an ideal position to observe unusual cases, develop rational explanations for the findings, and follow progress to determine if their hypotheses appear to be valid."[27]

Observation is indeed the key, for it leads to honest assessments of the merits and dangers of medications—to an appreciation of the individual nature of patients' responses and, therefore, the importance of individualizing treatment. Although physicians are taught to disdain "anecdotal" information, many important scientific discoveries began with incidental, unexpected findings by observant physicians.

This is why *Melmon and Morelli's Clinical Pharmacology: Basic Principles in Therapeutics* advises: "Only when the physician approaches each prescription as the beginning of a therapeutic experiment of uncertain outcome, and not as a concluding act to an office visit, will the chances that the experiment will be as safe, effective, and fruitful as possible be optimized."[28]

PHYSICIANS CAN ALSO play a pivotal role in rectifying many of the larger problems identified in this book. Patients need doctors, and drug companies need doctors. Doctors are the gatekeepers. They decide which drugs and dosages people receive, and in doing so they determine the success or failure of all medications. If doctors decide to reject a drug that is poorly researched or not properly dosed, the drug sells poorly and the manufacturer loses millions. If doctors decide to make cost a determining factor among similar drugs, drug prices will drop. Perhaps doctors do not have complete freedom of action, because they are responsible for choosing the best drug for each patient, but often there are choices between drugs that work similarly. Only rarely are doctors limited to one choice.

By reasserting their primary allegiance to their patients, doctors could pressure drug companies to produce better research, to provide more comprehensive information, and to manufacture medications with dosages designed to fit the widely varying needs of patients. Doctors could erase the growing feeling among patients that doctors today are mere "pill pushers," and instead reinvigorate their standing as scientists exercising their own independent knowledge and judgment in behalf of the well-being and safety of their patients.

In 2000, Catherine DeAngelis, the editor in chief of *JAMA,* wrote that physicians must "take back from business organizations the ultimate responsibility for patient care, the education of physicians, and new medical discovery."[29] A few physicians recognize that these changes are essential. In March 2001, I spoke with Dr. Drummond Rennie, an assistant editor at *JAMA* and a faculty member at the University of California, San Francisco, and also a leader in the effort to improve the quality of information from drug-company research. Dr. Rennie told me, "I get ten telephone calls a day from physicians concerned about these problems."

This is a nice start, but a couple thousand concerned doctors among 600,000 is still a small minority. It will take many more for physicians to reassert the scientific foundations of their profession, and in doing so to demand thorough research, complete and current information, and medications with dosages designed to fit patients and, thereby, to minimize the risks of side effects.

How Doctors Can Bridge the Patient-Doctor Divide and Revitalize the Medical System

1. Protest the side-effect epidemic: Doctors must insist that drug companies develop their medications based on sound medical principles with properly designed dosages and pills. Doctors can end the side-effect epidemic—if they make it a top priority.

2. Improve communication between doctors and patients: Many doctors are poor communicators. Medical schools must emphasize communication skills as a requirement for admission. Cooperative medicine must replace the old prescriptive model.

3. Expand medical training in medications: Current medical training about medications is grossly inadequate. Simplistic, cookbook methods are passed between generations of doctors, most of whom are reliant on drug-company guidelines. Advanced courses in clinical pharmacology should teach doctors to be independent thinkers, to read drug-company research critically, and to observe and handle patients' differing responses to medications.

4. Take all complaints of side effects seriously: There is no excuse for not checking a reliable drug reference before dismissing a patient's complaint. Doctors must move beyond their denial about side effects, relearning the value of independent observation and respecting the experiences of patients.

5. Provide informed consent: Informed consent is a basic principle of medical ethics. Patients are entitled to know why a drug is being prescribed and how the specific dose was selected. They are entitled to be told about side effects, long-term risks, as well as other options and other doses, especially lower, safer doses. There is no justification for withholding this information from patients.

6. Close the information gap: The drug-company–supported *PDR*, which is doctors' leading source of drug information, is not a complete drug reference. The practice of quality medicine depends on the availability of quality information. Doctors must demand that the drug companies produce a *PDR* that provides current and comprehensive information of high quality. Otherwise, as a profession, doctors should discourage the dissemination and wide acceptance of the *PDR*, and they should develop a reliable source of information of their own.

Chapter 14

How to Avoid Side Effects and Use Medications Safely

WITH 46 PERCENT of Americans taking at least one prescription drug daily, people must apply the same smart-shopping skills to their medications that they have developed for buying cars, clothing, and cosmetics. While people can usually rely on what a new car, cosmetic, or article of clothing will provide, whenever a person takes a medication for the first time, the outcome is never certain.

"The sad truth is that, even after all the clinical development that occurs with every drug and even after drugs have been approved for a time, we only have a crude idea of what they do in people," Dr. Janet Woodcock, director of the FDA's center for drug evaluation and research, told the *Los Angeles Times* in 1999.[1]

This is why you need to be as informed as possible. This chapter provides strategies for you to approach medication treatment with knowledge and preparedness, so that you can maximize your benefits and minimize your risks when using almost any medication.

Avoiding Side Effects Means
Getting the Right Dosage

Is it really important to match the dosage to the individual? Ask the family of Derek Smith, a talented professional basketball player whom I watched many times. In August 1996, while on a cruise with his wife and children and several teammates, Smith took a nonprescription drug for motion sickness. He developed acute respiratory failure and died. Smith was 34 years old, healthy, fit—and unusually sensitive to a common medication.

Stories like this are especially sad because they are so preventable. No matter how much we know about any drug, no matter whether the drug is obtained over-the-counter or by prescription, when you take it for the first time, it is an entirely new experiment. Everyone is different. That's why in using medications, individual variation isn't the exception, it's the rule. This means that whenever you or anyone else takes a medication for the first time, there is always an element of unpredictability and risk. This is why *Goodman and Gilman's The Pharmacological Basis of Therapeutics,* a highly respected pharmacology reference, states: "Any drug, no matter how trivial its therapeutic actions, has the potential to do harm."[2]

A drug may be "safe and effective" according to the FDA, but this term doesn't mean the drug may not harm some people. Even if the FDA were run by Ralph Nader, every drug it approved would still have some risks. Drug studies conducted with one or two thousand subjects can provide considerable information, but they cannot predict how millions of people of differing ages, sizes, states of health, and medication sensitivities will respond after the drug is approved. Nor can any study predict how any drug will affect any one person. However, it can be predicted that many people will respond to medication dosages lower than recommended by drug companies.

Always Start with the Lowest Effective Dosage Whenever Medically Possible

With any medication, you have two choices. You can take the higher, manufacturer-recommended initial dose, which may work fine or may cause side effects. Or you can start with the very lowest effective dose, such as the doses listed in "Lower, Safer Effective Doses for 53 Top-Selling Drugs" at the end of this chapter. These lower doses may work fine, or they may be too mild and will need to be increased.

The difference in approaches is simply this: taking the full dosage provides you with a more potent effect more quickly, at the cost of increased risks; the low-dose approach emphasizes safety, minimizes the risks and severity of side effects, and minimizes the rare, catastrophic reaction that occurred to Derek Smith, hundreds of men starting Viagra, and thousands of women taking the original high-dose birth control pills. In addition, for people taking medications long-term, the low-dose approach ensures that you receive only as much medication as you actually need, thereby reducing the risks of unforeseen, long-term side effects.

The obvious advantages of the low-dose approach are why my cardinal rule of medication usage is this:

> Except in emergencies or other acute situations, there usually is no reason to start with the full recommended dosage of most drugs. Always start with the lowest, safest, effective dose.

Unfortunately, finding information on lower effective doses isn't always easy. The drug descriptions in the *PDR* and other drug references contain a small amount of low-dose information. Medline and search engines such as Pubmed and Medscape offer more information, but it is usually difficult to find. The box section on page 248 offers the effective low doses of fifty-three major medications, but my research does not encompass all of the hundreds of frequently prescribed drugs in America. Thus, even if your drug reference doesn't mention a dose lower than a manufacturer recommends or you cannot find any low-dose studies in the medical literature, this doesn't mean that a lower dose doesn't work.

There are a few exceptions to the low-dose approach, such as in acute or severe conditions. Antibiotic or antifungal drugs should not be used at doses lower than manufacturers recommend, because lower doses may be too low to eradicate the infections. But for most conditions that doctors treat, the low-dose approach works well.

After I wrote my article in *Newsweek* (December 6, 1999), I received e-mails from around the country. One doctor wrote, "I just wanted to drop you a note saying how much I liked your article in *Newsweek*. I have always found that patients do well on low, 'subtherapeutic' doses, which are not 'just placebos.'" By "subtherapeutic," he meant doses that most doctors consider ineffective and not even worth trying. That is, doses lower than the drug companies recommend. Most doctors assume that any dose less than the manufacturer-recommended doses is ineffective, or subtherapeutic. This assumption is wrong.

Identifying Your Own Medication Sensitivity

People vary widely in their responses to biologically active chemicals, as seen every day in the different tolerances people exhibit to alcohol and coffee. But whereas people can find their own sensitivities to these drinks by sipping until they've had enough, with a pill it's all or nothing. That's why it's so important to use the dose that's right for you. "You run into patients all of the time who don't tolerate standard doses," Holly Whitcomb, the owner of four pharmacies in the Seattle area, told *Drug Therapy* for its 2000 article "Is Standard Dosing to Blame for Adverse Drug Reactions?"[3] Dr. Raymond Woosley, the chairman of the department of pharmacology at the Georgetown University Medical Center, added, "To think that the same dose will do the same thing to all patients is absurd. Patients need to be titrated, starting with the lowest possible dose that could have the desired effect."[4]

Finding the right dose rests on knowing your medication sensitivity. The questionnaire "Are You Sensitive to Medications?" (page 250), variations of which have been published in medical journals,[5] *The New York Times,*[6] and *Consumer Reports,*[7] can help you and your doctor gauge this. Your experience with alcohol, coffee, and other medications provides helpful clues. For example, if over-the-counter cold remedies or antihistamines make you sleepy, then prescription drugs that can cause sedation are likely to do the same. If coffee makes you edgy, then you may be prone to a similar reaction with Claritin-D or antidepressants like Prozac, Wellbutrin, Zoloft, or Paxil, or over-the-counter decongestants like Sudafed. Box sections on pages 252 and 254 list medications that may pose problems for people who are sensitive to the sedating or energizing effects of drugs.

Personal tendencies can also provide clues. For example, if you get light-headed when getting up too quickly, you may be prone to similar problems with drugs that reduce blood pressure such as Viagra, some muscle relaxants, and drugs for hypertension.

Family tendencies should also be considered. A specialist in women's medicine told me, "If their mothers are sensitive to a drug, many of my female patients are sensitive too." Family experiences may help in choosing between similar drugs. There are six cholesterol-lowering drugs, but if your brother has done well with Pravachol without side effects, you might do the same.

Size is also a factor, but it can be misleading. In a broad population, small people probably need lower doses more often, overall, than large people. However, some small people have high tolerances to medications, while some large people do not. One patient, who is over six feet tall and weighs more than 200 pounds, cannot tolerate the regular dosage of over-the-counter Sudafed, which dries out his system so powerfully, he develops constipation. So he takes half of the recommended dosage and still obtains the benefit without the problems.

Even with considerable information, your responses to medication can be unpredictable. Your degree of sensitivity can vary from drug to drug—even between drugs that have similar effects. One doctor I know gets depressed when he takes Motrin but does fine with Aleve.

Another does fine with Motrin but gets nauseated with Meclomen. Claritin makes one doctor sleepy (although Claritin is supposedly "non-sedating," it sedates 8 percent of users)[8] but Allegra doesn't.

One woman had such a bad reaction to Lilly's recommended initial dose of Prozac (20 mg/day), she avoided treatment for years. Yet, she ultimately did fine on Paxil. Indeed, she needed a moderately high dose, 30 mg/day. In contrast, when her friend took a low dose of Paxil (10 mg), the friend had to quit because of weight gain, a common although frequently overlooked side effect of these types of antidepressants.

Whereas most people encounter a medication sensitivity here or there, some people seem sensitive to just about everything. I call this a *general medication sensitivity*. My guess is that 5 to 10 percent of the population have general medication sensitivities, and that it occurs more frequently in women than men. One woman told me, "I react to everything. I don't know what will happen when the day comes that I really need treatment."

Her concern is warranted, because these patients are often switched from drug to drug to drug, encountering side effects each time and feeling miserable. A letter published in January 2001 in the "People's Pharmacy" column illustrated the problem perfectly:

> We visited my mother over the holidays, and she just isn't her old self. I'm convinced the problem is her medicine. She has been on Prozac, Paxil, Effexor, Zoloft, and Celexa. She has suffered from anxiety and restlessness, insomnia, dry mouth, and nausea. Her doctor is ready to give up. She is currently taking Remeron, but she is tired and dizzy all of the time. She has also gained weight.[9]

Medication sensitivities shouldn't be such a mystery. Science even has a name for such people: "poor metabolizers" (or "slow metabolizers"). These people simply cannot break down and eliminate drugs as quickly as others. A case report in a medical journal described the dilemma of one woman:

Over the years she had considerable difficulties in explaining to prescribing physicians that she was a slow metabolizer of antidepressants and its implications for drug dosage. After many problems with side effects on various antidepressants, she decided to drop all drug therapy. . . .[10]

Quitting treatment isn't an ideal solution. Understanding your medication sensitivities and possessing knowledge about lower, safer drug doses is the way to assure optimal care. "Both my mother and sister are very sensitive to medications," a woman told me. "Of course their doctors don't believe them, but they are very persistent and always demand the very lowest doses. Usually they get what they want."

Older People and Medication Sensitivities

Seventy-nine percent of all seniors take at least one prescription drug daily. Most people become increasingly sensitive to medications as they age, and medical conditions and multiple medications complicate the picture. Not coincidentally, the elderly experience the highest incidence of medication side effects, and the highest incidence of hospitalizations, disabilities, and deaths due to medications. The majority of these reactions are dose-related. Thus, the "Start low, go slow" approach applies especially to older people. Almost every expert recommends starting with very low doses with older people.

Yet, as discussed in Chapter 8, for scores of top-selling drugs, drug companies don't even bother to recommend lower doses for seniors. And because the drug companies don't recommend them, doctors don't consider prescribing lower doses, even for older people taking several other drugs. Therefore, the low-dose information in this book is especially important for older patients.

How Low Can You Go?

How low can a medication be started? Here's a case from one of the best drug references, the *United States Pharmacopoeia* (1994).[11] A woman had Mediterranean fever, a genetic disorder affecting protein production in the body and causing severe inflammation. By far, the best medication for Mediterranean fever is colchicine, a drug that is notorious for causing side effects. Colchicine causes stomach pain, cramping, and diarrhea in about 80 percent of patients. Of course, part of the problem is that colchicine is made in only one pill size, so even though these side effects are dose-related, using lower doses is difficult.

Colchicine made this woman very sick, but she had a creative physician who understood the principle of individual variation. He knew that if you start any person low enough, in time the person's system usually adjusts, and if you increase the medication slowly enough, you can usually reach an effective dosage. The doctor started this woman with the lowest medication dosage I have ever heard: .001 mg, which is 1/600 of the standard starting colchicine dose. He then increased the dose very gradually. Three months later the woman reached the full, necessary dosage she required.

If you start low enough and go slow enough, almost any person can be treated with any medication (assuming they are not allergic to it). I've had some patients start at one quarter and even one tenth the standard starting doses of drugs. With time, the dosage can usually be raised. Sometimes it isn't necessary, because very low doses are enough for some people. Even I was amazed at times, but then I realized that if drug responses can vary up to 4,000 percent from one person to the next, as the AMA indicates, then just about anything is possible.

For People Requiring Higher Doses

Although I emphasize using lower doses, not everyone responds to low-dose therapy. Some people need standard or even higher doses. One man wrote to me about his difficulties in getting enough medication. He weighs 350 pounds and is highly tolerant of medications. But just as doctors are reluctant to use doses below the manufacturers' recommendations, they are even more reluctant to go above these recommendations. Yet, we know from the principle of individual variation that just as some people are unusually sensitive to drugs, others, like this man, may be unusually unresponsive and require high doses. But just as a lot of low-dose information is omitted from standard drug references, so also is high-dose information.

For example, several people have told me that Claritin, the top-selling antihistamine, doesn't work for them. One woman said, "I miss Seldane [withdrawn in 1998 due to cardiac toxicities], because Claritin isn't nearly as good." She isn't alone. According to *The New York Times,* Schering's studies of Claritin at the recommended dosage of 10 mg produced improvement in less than 50 percent of patients, and the drug's performance was only slightly better than a placebo.[12] Dr. Sherwin Straus, the FDA officer reviewing Claritin, recommended a dose of 40 mg, but this dose would have required the listing of sedation as a side effect. Claritin's success rested on Schering's ability to market the drug as "nonsedating," so the dose was kept low—and less effective—to avoid this problem. The result is that many people who spend $80 to $100 for a month's supply of Claritin obtain little benefit. This might not be a problem if Schering informed physicians and patients that higher doses may sometimes be needed. Instead, with one-size-fits-all 10-mg Claritin (except for people with liver or kidney disease), some people receive only one half or one quarter the dose they actually require, but physicians are reluctant to prescribe higher doses—or lower doses—without any guidelines.

Ultimately it doesn't matter whether you need a low dose or high dose—what matters is that you are taking the right dose. But even if you need a higher dose of a medication, starting low and increasing gradually remains a good policy, because it triggers fewer side effects than starting with a high dose. I have seen this many times. Neurontin, which is used for pain syndromes and seizures, is recommended at 300 mg four times a day, but many people get light-headed or sedated or develop mental confusion at this standard dosage. Fortunately, Neurontin is also made in a 100-mg dose. If people start with this lower dose and then increase gradually, they have far fewer problems. I know people who ultimately required doses of 2,400 to 3,600 mg of Neurontin, but by starting low they encountered few difficulties.

Increasing the Dosage Safely

Most side effects occur with the first doses or when doses are increased. When drug companies recommend jumps in dosage of 100 percent, it is guaranteed to cause problems for some people. Even jumps of 50 percent may be too high for medication-sensitive people. Just because Pfizer says Lipitor should be dosed at 10–20–40 mg, it doesn't mean you must follow that regimen. Perhaps 15 mg is your ideal dose. Or 30 mg.

One man with chronic depression was desperate when 60 mg of Prozac, which had made him feel normal for the first time in his life, began causing serious side effects. Dropping to the next lowest recommended dose, 40 mg, caused a return of his depression. Back and forth he went from 60 mg to 40 mg to 60 mg to 40 mg, suffering each day. Yet, his doctor never considered the obvious, 50 mg, because the standard, drug-company-recommended protocol for Prozac is 20–40–60–80 mg. When adjusting drug doses, think creatively, and ask your doctor to think creatively too.

Tell your doctor to increase the dosage as gradually as possible. Sometimes doing it gradually is difficult because drug companies don't produce enough pill sizes or the drug only comes as a capsule. When a choice between medications exists, ask your doctor to prescribe drugs that allow flexible dosing.

Maintenance Doses Can Often Be Lower

If you will be taking medication for many months or years, it may be possible to reduce your dosage once your condition is well controlled. Although this isn't always possible, lower doses often suffice for maintenance treatment.

Unfortunately, doctors often do not try to lower the maintenance doses once acute conditions are controlled. In a National Institutes of Health study, researchers found that patients with a severe ulcerative condition could have their doses of Prilosec reduced by 50 to 75 percent, saving up to $4,000 annually.[13] These patients had been in treatment for one to two years; yet, their own physicians hadn't tried to reduce their high doses of Prilosec, a drug with unknown long-term effects. Indeed, a few years after Prilosec was approved, studies showed that it markedly reduced the absorption of vitamin B_{12}.[14] The stomach-acid–suppressing effect of Prilosec is dose-related, so the higher the Prilosec dosage, the greater the risk of B_{12} deficiency, which can cause serious problems.

Just as it is important to go slowly when increasing medication doses, it is equally important to go slowly when decreasing them. For example, if you are taking 40 mg of Prozac and want to try lowering it, the standard approach would be to drop to 20 mg/day, a sudden reduction of 50 percent. This is too much too quickly for some people. Lowering to 30 mg first allows a smoother transition with less likelihood of rebound or withdrawal reactions. Some medications, such as Xanax and Paxil, commonly cause reactions if decreased too rapidly.[15–17]

If you and your doctor agree to reduce your dosage, but your condition flares up, don't be discouraged. You may just need to reduce more gradually. Or you may already be at your ideal dosage, which you have now confirmed by your poor response to a lower dose. Some patients get fixated on lowering their dosage. Avoid this, because the goal is to take the amount you need.

Once Daily vs. Twice Daily, and Other Dosing Regimens

Drug companies are producing many new drugs with once-daily dosing regimens. Doctors like once-daily drugs, because they have been convinced that patients find it easier to remember to take once-daily pills. This is true—to a point—but sometimes there is a downside.

The problem with once-daily dosing is that you are socking your system with your entire day's dosage at one time. If you normally drink a cup of coffee in the morning, at lunch, and after dinner, what would happen if instead you drank all three cups at breakfast? It does save time and is easier to remember to do something once daily rather than several times a day, but your risks of getting edgy or anxious would increase greatly. To reduce the impact of once-daily drugs, pharmaceutical companies produce sustained-release pills that are supposed to dissolve gradually in the intestines. Sometimes this works, but some sustained-release pills do not dissolve evenly and exert most of their effects within a few hours of usage. This may be a problem for some people.

A few drugs, such as Norvasc and Serzone, are slowly absorbed and slowly metabolized, so that a once-dally dose provides a fairly even effect over twenty-four hours. With other drugs, however, a twice-daily regimen may sometimes be preferable to a once-daily one. Splitting the dosage over a day can reduce side effects, and taking pills twice daily isn't any more difficult to remember. People remember to take their medications if the dosing is combined with other regular activities. With twice-daily dosing, people take their medications with breakfast and with dinner. This is easy to remember. The greatest problems seem to occur with drugs that require three or four doses daily. Even so, in some situations, spreading a drug between three or four doses may further reduce side-effect risks.

You know the once-daily dosing trend has gone too far when drugs that work better twice daily are nonetheless marketed with once-daily regimens. For Aceon, a new antihypertensive drug, twice-daily dosing proved superior in tests,[18] but the drug is still advertised as "Once-Daily Aceon."

When Side Effects Occur

Although a "Start low, go slow" approach may greatly lower the risks of side effects, some adverse reactions will still occur. Medications are powerful chemicals, and some reactions cannot be anticipated.

Common side effects are usually easy to recognize. Most drug references provide lists of the most common side effects in early research. However, these references usually do not point out the dose-related nature of most side effects, so many doctors prescribe one drug after another without ever thinking about adjusting the dosage. The appropriate way to deal with a medication side effect is to simply lower the dosage or to switch to another drug at a low, safe dosage that is less likely to provoke problems.

Getting your physician's attention is another matter. Some physicians seem indifferent to so-called "minor" side effects such as headaches, abdominal pain, fatigue, ringing in the ears, joint pain, insomnia, constipation, and hundreds of others that make people miserable. Minor side effects not only diminish people's quality of life, but also cause millions to quit vital treatment for serious, life-shortening conditions such as high cholesterol or high blood pressure. Sometimes patients feel self-conscious about telling their doctors about these types of side effects. Be sure to let your doctor know about any side effect that is uncomfortable or alters normal functioning.

Patients frequently encounter problems when experiencing side effects that physicians don't recognize. In this situation you should check drug references at your bookstore and library to find mention of your problem. Copy the page, circle the side effect, and show it to your doctor. Documented information from a reliable source provides strong substantiation of your point of view.

The greatest difficulty for patients is when side effects—either because they are rare or because they weren't discovered until after the drug received FDA approval—are not listed in any drug references. This is not an uncommon occurrence, and getting your doctor's attention can be very difficult. You may have to broaden your search by using the Medscape or PubMed search engines on the Internet, or by going to a medical library to obtain assistance from a trained librarian. The Internet also has hundreds of Web sites formed by patients with medication reactions that their physicians ignored. Some Web sites provide a lot of information, but you must be selective. It is particularly helpful when Web sites list published articles in medical journals or the names of physicians who recognize these side effects and will treat patients experiencing them.

You might also show your doctor the following comments from Dr. Robert Fenichel, an officer at the FDA for eleven years and a deputy division director from 1996 until retiring in 2000. In a March 2001 interview with Denise Grady of *The New York Times*, Dr. Fenichel defined the limitations of research in identifying side effects: "If you have 3,000 patients . . . and something on average will occur [once] in 1,000 times in people using the drug, it is 95% likely that you will see such a thing in those 3,000 patients. Five percent of the time, you won't see this thing."[19] Five percent represents thousands of side effects when drugs are prescribed to millions of people. That's thousands of side effects that aren't recognized or listed anywhere.

With even rarer side effects, recognition is even less certain. Dr. Fenichel explained, "If something is happening in 1 in every 5,000, your chance of seeing it is pretty small. . . . Most things are very difficult to detect. And that means plenty of small effects will never be detected."[20] This is why it is so important for physicians and consumers to understand the shortcomings of drug-company research and the deficiencies in the information provided by drug-company advertising, sales representatives, package inserts, and *PDR* descriptions. This is why physicians must reacquaint themselves with the principle of individual variation in medication response, and must develop a better way of obtaining current, comprehensive information about medication doses and side effects.

When Your Drug Loses Effectiveness

Sometimes, after you have been on a medication for a while, it may seem to lose its effectiveness. Many patients conclude that they have become "immune" to the drugs' effects, and their doctors begin switching to other drugs, which raises new risks.

In my experience, when drugs become less effective, it is merely because of changes in the person's system. Most often, your body has simply become more efficient in metabolizing and eliminating the drug, so the drug's effect is reduced. People who drink coffee or alcohol every day usually develop some tolerance, because the body has become similarly efficient.

With medications, a slight upward adjustment in the dosage usually solves the problem. Ask your doctor, but my inclination has always

242

been that if a drug was working well, it is better to adjust its dosage to regain its effect rather than switch to other drugs that may not work as well or may cause side effects.

Stopping Medications Without Withdrawal Reactions

It seems elementary that if your body has depended on a medication for a while, abruptly discontinuing the drug might create problems. This doesn't happen with every drug, but it occurs fairly often. The drug companies and medical profession didn't recognize this issue for decades, but a large number of case reports about withdrawal reactions with antidepressants such as Paxil have led to wider recognition of the problem.[21-25] Withdrawal reactions are also common with sleep medications and drugs for anxiety. Abrupt reduction or discontinuation of antihypertensive medication can cause a rebound in blood pressure. Withdrawal syndromes can include lethargy, irritability, headaches, nausea, depression, or other symptoms.

Withdrawal reactions sometimes occur with drugs not generally associated with these problems. One report described a woman who became psychotic after stopping birth-control pills.[26] As every woman knows, changes in hormone levels can affect emotions. In this rare case, the abrupt discontinuation of birth-control pills produced a severe reaction.

Withdrawal reactions are not the rule, but they occur frequently and unpredictably enough to warrant consideration when stopping a medication you have taken regularly for a while. Ask your doctor if there are any withdrawal problems associated with the drug and whether it may be wiser to stop the drug gradually rather than abruptly.

New Drugs: Proceed with Caution

As discussed in Chapter 4, an Associated Press article in December 2000 quoted both Dr. Raymond Woosley and Dr. Jane Henney, then the commissioner of the FDA, as recommending caution in using newly approved drugs. "I sure wouldn't," Dr. Woosley said. "I don't personally, and I don't usually prescribe it unless I have to."

This is good advice, but what does this say about the safety, or lack of it, with new medications? When you think about it, these statements are testimony to the inadequacy of pre-release research by drug companies and the review process of the FDA. If new drugs aren't safe enough for experts like Dr. Woosley to consider, should anyone? If new drugs possess such dangers, shouldn't they be approved for limited usage and followed with careful monitoring?

Avoiding new drugs may be an option for some people, but what about the larger society? If these drugs are used only by the uninformed and by those who absolutely need the new drugs, aren't they being placed at unfair risk? Are they receiving proper consent? Proper monitoring?

Melmon and Morrelli's Clinical Pharmacology states: "It would disappoint the patients and the profession to realize how truly little of the important medical consequences is known about a new clinical entity [new drug] at the time it becomes a salable product."[27] This was written in 1993. With ten new drugs withdrawn between 1997 and 2000, this situation has clearly not improved.

Dr. Sidney Wolfe, who is the editor of Public Citizen's *Worst Pills, Best Pills News* and who follows FDA activities closely, is so skeptical of our current methods that he tells people to wait for five years before trying some new drugs. While I certainly recommend caution, I don't always agree with Dr. Wolfe. Sometimes, new drugs offer important advantages over older drugs. For example, Dr. Wolfe applies his five-year rule to Celebrex and Vioxx, the new anti-inflammatory drugs. I disagree, because older anti-inflammatory drugs cause thousands of deaths and tens of thousands of hospitalizations each year due to abdominal hemorrhaging. Celebrex and Vioxx appear to cause substantially fewer of these problems.

I would note that people doing fine with Motrin, Voltaren, or other anti-inflammatory drugs shouldn't automatically switch to these newer and much more expensive alternatives, but for the millions of

244

people who have problems with the older anti-inflammatories, Cele-brex and Vioxx may make a big difference in pain reduction and in-creased function. Most gastrointestinal and other side effects with anti-inflammatory drugs are dose-related, so using the lowest effective dose is still essential. Vioxx is easier to adjust than Celebrex, because Vioxx is made as a breakable tablet.

The bottom line with new medications is that unless there's a rea-son to switch to a new drug, don't. If a new drug must be used, the "Start low, go slow" approach should be considered.

Coping with Drug-Company Advertising

The billions spent for drug-company advertising are having their in-tended effect. People who never considered taking medication have gone to their physicians seeking it. In some respects, this is good, for it has motivated people needing treatment to finally get it. However, many of these people are asking for the drugs they've seen adver-tised—sometimes they are demanding them—and doctors are oblig-ing, sometimes unwisely.

If a drug-company advertisement catches your eye, there's nothing wrong in asking your doctor about the medication. Keep in mind, however, that the advertisement isn't giving you even half of the story. Ask your doctor if the advertisement is accurate. Is the advertised drug the correct one for you? What is its downside? Are there other al-ternatives that may be better, safer, or cheaper? Drug-company ads typically promote expensive brand-name products, although other drugs may be equally effective, more extensively studied, and less costly.

Do not assume that if a drug is advertised, it is not side-effect prone. In 1999, the maker of Fosamax aired advertisements directed toward women concerned about osteoporosis. Fosamax does prevent this serious weakening of the bones, but it is so caustic, it frequently causes heartburn, and cases have been reported of severe irritations and erosions of the esophagus requiring hospitalization and surgery. A January 2001 article in the *Archives of Internal Medicine* found that just ten days of Fosamax led to gastric irritation in 33 percent and gastric ulcers in 7 percent of patients.[28] When used with an anti-inflammatory drug, 38 percent developed ulcers. With the long-term usage that is required with Fosamax, even higher numbers of ulcers can be expected.

Just as you don't go out and buy a car based solely on its advertising, don't seek a medication based on its advertising. Get objective information. Go to the library or bookstore. Check the Internet Web sites of respected institutions and Web sites for people reporting reactions to the drug. Ask your doctor and pharmacist. Information is power. In today's medical-pharmaceutical complex, you need as much information as you can get.

How to Obtain Informed Consent— And Your Doctor's Cooperation

The American Medical Association Council on Ethical and Judicial Affairs states that you have "a right to receive information from physicians and to discuss the benefits, risks, and costs of appropriate treatment alternatives." This right exists "only if the patient possesses enough information to enable an intelligent choice. The physician's obligation is to present the medical facts accurately to the patient or to the individual responsible for the patient's care and to make recommendations for management in accordance with good medical practice. The physician has an ethical obligation to help the patient make choices from among the therapeutic alternatives consistent with good medical practice."[29]

Informed consent may be your basic right, but some rights exist in theory more than they do in practice. Studies have shown that when doctors prescribe medications, few patients receive adequate informed consent. One study videotaping interactions between physicians and patients found that 91 percent of these interactions failed to meet the requirements of informed decision making.[30] Today, with doctors having less time than ever to communicate with patients, obtaining informed consent is even more difficult. This is regrettable because, as reported by the *British Medical Journal* in February 2001, "Patients in primary care strongly want a patient centered approach with communication, partnership, and health promotion."[31]

Fortunately, people are becoming more assertive about their medical care. This is a very positive step, but good, *objective* information is still hard to find. You have a difficult task. My advice is: Read, ask, think. Use all reasonable resources, including books, medical journals, and the Web sites of respected institutions and experts, as well as Web sites of patients who present credible information. In my experience, the best drug reference is the *American Hospital Formulary Service*.[32] It provides a great deal of in-depth information, but it is costly and written for professionals.

Scientifically based information is a powerful tool. Your ideas may be worthwhile, but your doctor is a scientist, and he is trained to be skeptical of anything not scientifically validated. This is why many physicians are disdainful of stories from patients and unsubstantiated information from the Internet. Your job, therefore, is to find dependable information that, when necessary, you can show your physician. When you place a drug reference or a journal article or a pile of abstracts on your doctor's desk, it will get his attention.

I HAVE NEVER KNOWN a person who liked taking medications. I have never known a person who, having to take medication, wanted to take a milligram more than absolutely necessary. Patients are concerned about the risks with medications, especially the risks that occur with higher doses, even if the drug companies are not. My goal in writing *Over Dose* is to provide you with informed consent about the unacceptable state of medication treatment today, and to empower you with specific information about how to obtain the very lowest, safest medication doses that you require. By doing so, my aim is to reduce your risks—and to begin to end the side-effect epidemic. The current system of inadequate dosage research and unsound prescribing methods will change only when you and millions of others understand the fundamental problems and demand change.

As I said at the beginning of this book, I am pro-medication. We have many highly effective drugs today, and even better drugs will soon begin arriving as a result of breakthroughs involving the genetic code, cloning, and other advanced techniques. Even with these amazing advances, however, individual variation will remain a major factor in determining how you respond to medications. Until the drug companies and other participants in the health-care system dedicate their efforts to producing medications that fit people, the side-effect epidemic will continue, and it will be up to you to protect yourself and your loved ones. With the information in this book, and from all of the other resources available today, you have the power to demand intelligent, scientifically based treatment—and to maximize the benefits and minimize the risks of any medications you take.

Lower, Safer, Effective Doses for 53 Top-Selling Drugs That You Won't Find in the PDR or Most Other Drug References

MEDICATION	DRUG COMPANY INITIAL DOSAGE	EFFECTIVE, LOWER INITIAL DOSAGE
Aldactone (spironolactone)	50–100 mg/day	25 mg
Allegra (fexofenadine)	60 mg twice daily	20 mg three times a day or 40 mg twice daily
Altace (ramipril)	2.5 mg/day	1.25 mg/day
Ambien (zolpidem)	10 mg	5 mg or 7.5 mg at bedtime
Axid (nizatidine)	150 mg twice daily or 300 mg at bedtime	25–75 mg twice daily or 100 mg at bedtime
Baycol (cerivastatin)	0.4 mg/day	0.2 or 0.3 mg/day
Calan (verapamil)	120–180 mg/day	90 mg/day
Celebrex (celecoxib)	100 mg twice daily	50 mg twice daily
Cozaar (losartan)	50 mg/day	25 mg/day
Cytotec (misoprostol)	200 mcg four times a day	50 or 100 mcg four times a day
Dalmane (flurazepam)	30 mg at bedtime	15 mg at bedtime
Demadex (torsemide)	10 mg/day	5 mg/day
Desyrel (trazodone)	150 mg/day	25–100 mg/day
Dyrenium (triamterene)	100 mg twice daily	25–100 mg daily
Edecrin (ethacrynic acid)	50 mg/day	25 mg/day
Effexor (venlafaxine)	75 mg/day	37.5 or 50 mg/day
Elavil (amitriptyline)	50–75 mg/day	10–25 mg/day
Estrace (oral estradiol)	1–2 mg/day	0.5 mg/day
Estraderm (transdermal estradiol)	0.05–0.1 mg/day	0.02–0.025 mg/day
Estratab (esterified estrogens)	1.25 mg/day	0.3–0.625 mg/day
Hydrochlorothiazide (HCTZ)	25 mg/day	12.5 mg/day
Hygroton (chlorthalidone)	15 mg/day	12.5 mg/day
Inderal (propranolol) (regular and XL)	80 mg/day	40 mg/day
Isoptin (verapamil)	120–180 mg/day	90 mg/day
Lasix (furosemide)	80 mg/day	40 mg/day
Levatol (penbutolol)	10 mg/day	20 mg/day*
Lipitor (atorvastatin)	10 mg/day	2.5 or 5 mg/day
Lopressor (metoprolol)	50–100 mg/day	50 mg/day**
Mevacor (lovastatin)	20 mg/day	10 mg/day
Motrin (ibuprofen)	300–400 mg three or four times a day	200 mg three times a day
Norvasc (amlodipine)	5 mg/day	2.5 mg/day***
Pamelor (nortriptyline)	50–75 mg/day	10 or 25 mg/day

Pepcid (famotidine)	20 mg twice daily or 40 mg at bedtime	10 mg twice daily or 20 mg at bedtime
Plendil (felodipine)	5 mg/day	2.5 mg/day
Pravachol (pravastatin)	10–20 mg/day	5–10 mg/day
Premarin (conjugated estrogens), for vasomotor symptoms or osteoporosis	0.625 mg/day	0.3 mg/day
Prilosec (omeprazole)	20 mg/day	10 mg/day
Privinil (lisinopril)	10 mg/day	5 mg/day
Prozac (fluoxetine)	20 mg/day	2.5, 5, or 10 mg/day
Sectral (acebutolol)	400 mg/day	200 mg/day
Serzone (nefazodone)	100 mg twice daily	50 mg daily or twice daily
Sinequan (doxepin)	75 mg/day	10, 25, or 50 mg/day
Tagamet (cimetidine)	800 mg at bedtime	400 mg at bedtime
Tenormin (atenolol)	50 mg/day	25 mg/day
Tofranil (imipramine)	75 mg/day	10–25 mg/day
Verelan (verapamil)	120–180 mg/day	90 mg/day
Voltaren (diclofenac)	50 mg two, three, or four times a day	25 mg three times a day
Wellbutrin (bupropion)	100 mg twice daily	50 mg twice daily
Zantac (ranitidine)	150 mg twice daily or 300 mg at bedtime	100 mg twice daily
Zebeta (bisoprolol)	5 mg/day	2.5 mg/day****
Zestril (lisinopril)	10 mg/day	5 mg/day
Zocor (simvastatin)	10–20 mg/day	2.5, 5, or 10 mg/day
Zofran (ondansetron)	8 mg twice daily	1–4 mg three times a day
Zoloft (setraline)	50 mg/day	25 mg/day

*The *PDR* states, "A dose of 10 mg also lowers blood pressure, but the full effect is not seen for 4–8 weeks."

**One brand of metoprolol is recommended at 100 mg/day initially, whereas another brand is recommended at 50–100 mg/day.

***The *PDR*'s "usual" initial dose of Norvasc is 5 mg/day, but then it adds that 2.5 mg may be sufficient for small, elderly, or debilitated patients. Experts recommend 2.5 mg initially for all patients.

****The *PDR*'s "usual" initial dose of bisoprolol is 5 mg/day, but it adds that 2.5 mg may be sufficient for "some patients." JNC VI recommends 2.5 mg initially for all patients.

Adapted from: Cohen, J. S. "Dose Discrepancies between the *Physicians' Desk Reference* and the Medical Literature, and Their Possible Relationship to the Incidence of Adverse Drug Events." *Archives of Internal Medicine,* April 2001; 161: 957–64.

This listing is for information purposes only. Readers should not change drugs or dosages unless specifically directed to do so by their own doctors.

Are You Sensitive to Medications?

For You And Your Doctor When Deciding On Medications*

1. Are you sensitive to any prescription or nonprescription drugs? If yes, please list and describe:

2. How are you affected by alcohol? Check one and describe:
_____ Easily affected _____ Moderately affected _____ Not affected

3. Do some drugs make you tired or sleepy? If so, please list and describe:

Cold or allergy remedies or antihistamines (such as Benadryl, Claritin, Contac, Tavist, Zyrtec, etc.):

Benzodiazepines (tranquilizers or anticonvulsants, such as Ativan, Klonopin, Valium, Xanax):

Others (such as motion-sickness remedies Dramamine or Bonine, or antinausea agents Phenergan or Compazine):

4. Do some drugs give you energy, or cause anxiety or insomnia? If so, please list and describe:

Coffee, tea, or other caffeine-containing substances:

Appetite suppressants (prescription or nonprescription):

Cold or allergy remedies or decongestants (such as Sudafed):

Others:

5. Have you ever had a reaction to epinephrine (adrenaline chloride, often injected by dentists with pain-numbing medication)? Typical reactions include palpitations, sweating, anxiety, and headaches:

6. Have you had any side effects (such as impaired memory or coordination, blurred vision, headaches, indigestion, diarrhea, constipation, dizziness, palpitations, rashes, swelling, ringing in the ears, other reactions) from any other prescription or nonprescription drugs? If so, please list the drugs and briefly describe side effects:

7. Overall, how would you describe yourself with regard to medications?

____ Very sensitive

____ Not particularly sensitive to medications

____ Very tolerant, usually require high doses

*Adapted from: Cohen, J.S. "Ways To Minimize Adverse Drug Reactions: Individualized Doses and Common Sense Are Key." *Postgraduate Medicine,* Sept. 1999;106:163-72.

Medications That Can Cause Sedation

If you are sensitive to medications that cause sedation, drowsiness, or fatigue, you should avoid the drugs listed here. If they must be used, they should be used at very low doses initially.

Antihistamines:

Benadryl (diphenhydramine)

Dramamine (dimenhydrinate)

Antivert, Bonine, Dramamine II (meclizine)

Marezine (cyclizine)

Atarax, Vistaril (hydroxyzine)

Tavist (clemastine)

Other nonprescription cold, cough, allergy, sinus, and sleep remedies that contain antihistamines.

Anti-Anxiety Medications: All may cause sedation, but these may be particularly sedating to sedation-prone individuals:

Valium (diazepam)

Serax (oxazepam)

Klonopin (clonazepam)

Ativan (lorazepam)

Sleep Remedies: All prescription (e.g., Halcion, Dalmane, Ambien) and nonprescription (e.g., Sominex) sleep remedies may produce increased and/or prolonged effects in susceptible individuals.

Antidepressants: Those frequently causing sedation include:

Elavil (amitriptyline)

Adapin, Sinequan (doxepin)

Desyrel (trazodone)

Paxil (paroxetine)

Ludiomil (maprotiline)

Beta Blockers: All may cause drowsiness or lethargy in susceptible individuals, including Inderal, Tenormin, Lopressor.

Prescription Pain Remedies containing opiates such as codeine, Percodan, Percocet, Vicodin.

Phenothiazines: All may cause sedation, but these may be particularly sedating to sedation-sensitive individuals:

Phenergan (promethazine): Frequently used for motion sickness and nausea.

Thorazine (chlorpromazine)

Mellaril (thioridazine)

Muscle Relaxants:

Flexeril (cyclobenzaprine)

Parafon Forte (chlorzoxazone)

Soma (carisoprodol)

Robaxin (methocarbamol)

Medications That Can Cause Nervousness, Agitation, or Insomnia

If you are sensitive to medications that cause edginess, nervousness, anxiety, or insomnia, you should avoid the drugs listed here. If they must be used, they should be taken at very low doses initially.

Decongestants: The most common decongestant used in nonprescription cold, cough, and sinus remedies is pseudoephedrine. Well-known preparations containing decongestants are Sudafed, Drixoral, Afrin, and non-drowsy formulas of Contac, Allerest, Sinarest, and many others. These and similar drugs can cause edginess or agitation in medication-sensitive individuals.

Antidepressants: Some antidepressants can cause anxiety, agitation, or insomnia even in people not prone to these symptoms.

Prozac (fluoxetine)

Zoloft (sertraline)

Paxil (paroxetine)

Wellbutrin (bupropion)

Effexor (venlafaxine)

Tofranil (imipramine)

Norpramin (desipramine)

Vivactil (protriptyline)

Nardil (phenelzine)

Diet Pills: Most prescription (except Pondimin) and nonprescription diet pills.

Ritalin (methylphenidate)

Phenothiazines: Although the mechanism is different from direct stimulants, some phenothiazines are prone to causing agitation-like symptoms.

Compazine (prochlorperazine): frequently used for nausea

Haldol (haloperidol)

Stelazine (trifluoperazine)

Prolixin (fluphenazine)

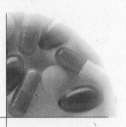

References

Chapter 1

1. Wernicke, J.F., Dunlop, S.R., Dornseif, B.E., Bosomworth, J.C., and Humbert, M. "Low-dose fluoxetine therapy for depression." *Psychopharmacology Bulletin,* 1988; 24(1):183–188.

2. Louie, A.K., Lewis, T.B., and Lannon, M.D. "Use of low-dose fluoxetine in major depression and panic disorder." *Journal of Clinical Psychiatry,* 1993; 54(1):435–438.

3. Lazarou, J., Pomeranz, B.H., and Corey, P.N. "Incidence of adverse drug reactions in hospitalized patients: a meta-analysis of prospective studies [see comments]." *JAMA,* April 15, 1998, 279(15):1200–5.

4. *Ibid.*

5. Gilman, A.G., Rall, T.W., Nies, A.S., and Taylor, P. *Goodman and Gilman's The Pharmacological Basis of Therapeutics.* New York: Pergamon Press, 1990 and 1996.

6. Kolata, G. (New York Times News Service). "Who cares when our drugs fail?" *San Diego Union-Tribune,* Wed., Oct. 15, 1997:E-1,5.

7. Melmon, K.L., Morrelli, H.F., Hoffman, B.B., and Nierenberg, D.W. *Melmon and Morrelli's Clinical Pharmacology: Basic Principles in Therapeutics* (3rd edition). New York: McGraw-Hill, Inc., 1993.

8. Moore, T.J., Psaty, B.M., and Furberg, C.D. "Time to act on drug safety." *JAMA,* May 20, 1998, 279(19):1571–3.

9. Cullen, D.J., Bates, D.W., Small, S.D., Cooper, J.B., Nemeskal, A.R., and Leape, L.L. "The incident reporting system does not detect adverse drug events: a problem for quality improvement." *Joint Commission Journal on Quality Improvement,* Oct. 1995, 21(10): 541–8.

10. Bates, D.W. "Drugs and adverse drug reactions: how worried should we be?" *JAMA,* April 15, 1998, 279(15):1216–7.

11. Dickinson, J.G. *Dickinson's FDA Review,* March 2000; 7(3):13–14.

12. Marks, L. "Not just a statistic": the history of USA and UK policy over thrombotic disease and the oral contraceptive pill, 1960s–1970s. *Social Science and Medicine,* 1999 Nov, 49(9):1139–55.

13. Van Hoften, C., Burger, H., Peeters, P.H., Grobbee, D.E., Van Noord, P.A., Leufkens, H.G. "Long-term oral contraceptive use increases breast cancer risk in women over 55 years of age: the DOM cohort." *International Journal of Cancer,* 2000;87(4):591–4.

14. Burke, W. "Oral Contraceptives and Breast Cancer." *JAMA,* Oct. 11, 2000; 284:1837–38.

15. Schlesselman, J.J. "Net effect of oral contraceptive use on the risk of cancer in women in the United States." *Obstetrics and Gynecology,* 1995 May, 85(5 Pt 1):793–801.

16. Bagshaw, S. "The Combined Oral Contraceptive." *Drug Safety,* 1995; 12:91–96.

17. Ettinger, B. "Personal perspective on low-dosage estrogen therapy for postmenopausal women." *Menopause,* 1999; 6(3):273–6.

18. Weinstein, L. "Efficacy of a continuous estrogen-progestin regimen in the menopausal patient." *Obstetrics and Gynecology,* 1987; 69(6):929–32.

19. Greendale, G.A., Reboussin, B.A., Hogan, P., Barnabei, V.M., Shumaker, S., Johnson, S., et al. "Symptom relief and side effects

of postmenopausal hormones: results from the Postmenopausal Estrogen/Progestin Interventions Trial." *Obstetrics and Gynecology,* 1998;92(6):982–8.

20. Ettinger B. op. cit.

21. American Society of Hospital Pharmacists. American Hospital Formulary Service, Drug Information 1999. Gerald K. McEvoy, Editor. Bethesda, MD: 1999.

22. American Medical Association. AMA Drug Evaluations, Annual 1993. Chicago: American Medical Association, 1993.

23. Lindsay, R., Hart, D.M., Clark, D.M. "The minimum effective dose of estrogen for prevention of postmenopausal bone loss." *Obstetrics and Gynecology,* 1984;63(6):759–63.

24. Ettinger, B. "A practical guide to preventing osteoporosis." *Western Journal of Medicine,* 1988;149(6):691–5.

25. Schairer, C., Lubin, J., Troisi, R., Sturgeon, S., Brinton, L., Hoover, R. "Menopausal estrogen and estrogen-progestin replacement therapy and breast cancer risk." *JAMA,* 2000 Jan 26, 283(4):485–91.

26. Persson, I., Weiderpass, E., Bergkvist, L., Bergstrom, R., Schairer, C. "Risks of breast and endometrial cancer after estrogen and estrogen-progestin replacement." *Cancer Causes and Control,* 1999 Aug, 10(4):253–60.

27. Peck, C., Barr, W., Benet, L., Collins, J., Desjardins, R., Furst, D., et al. "Opportunities for integrating of pharmacokinetics, pharmacodynamics, and toxicokinetics in rational drug development." *Journal of Clinical Pharmacology,* 1994; 34:111–19.

28. Peck, C.C. "Drug development: improving the process." *Food Drug Law Journal,* 1997, 52:163–7.

29. Woosley, R.L. "Drug Labeling Revisions—Guaranteed to Fail?" *JAMA,* Dec. 20, 2000, 284(23):3047–49.

30. Sussman, N. "More Questions Than Answers." *Primary Psychiatry,* 2000, 7:6.

31. Angell, M. "The Pharmaceutical Industry—To Whom Is It Accountable?" *The New England Journal of Medicine,* 2000, 342: 1902–4.

32. Melmon et al., op. cit.

33. Bowman, L. "51% Of U.S. Adults Take 2 Pills or More a Day, Survey Reports" (Scripps Howard News Service). *San Diego Union-Tribune,* Wed., Jan. 17, 2001, A8.

34. Cullen et al., op. cit.

35. Gilman et al., op. cit.

36. Cohen, J.S. and Insel, P.A. "The Physicians' Desk Reference. Problems and possible improvements." *Archives of Internal Medicine,* 1996, 156(13):1375–80.

37. Cohen, J.S. "Adverse drug effects, compliance, and the initial doses of antihypertensive drugs recommended by the Joint National Committee vs. the Physicians' Desk Reference." *Archives of Internal Medicine,* 2001, 161:880–85.

38. Cohen, J.S. "Dose Discrepancies between the Physicians' Desk Reference and the Medical Literature, and Their Possible Role in the High Incidence of Dose-Related Adverse Drug Events." *Archives of Internal Medicine,* April 9, 2001. Scheduled for publication.

39. Cohen, J.S. "Ways To Minimize Adverse Drug Reactions: Individualized Doses and Common Sense Are Key." *Postgraduate Medicine,* Sept. 1999, 106:163–72.

40. Cohen, J.S. "Adverse Drug Reactions: Effective Low-Dose Therapies for Older Patients." *Geriatrics,* Feb. 2000, 55(2):54–64.

41. Cohen, J.S. "Comparison of FDA Reports of Patient Deaths Associated with Sildenafil (Viagra) and with Injectable Alprostadil." *Annals of Pharmacotherapy,* March 2001, 35:285–88.

42. Cohen, J.S. "Is the Product Information on Sildenafil (Viagra) Adequate to Facilitate Optimal Therapeutics and to Minimize Adverse Events?" *Annals of Pharmacotherapy,* March 2001, 35: 337–42.

43. Cohen, J.S. "Should Patients Be Given a Low Test Dose of Viagra Initially?" *Drug Safety,* July 2000, 23:1–10.

44. Rennie, D. "Fair Conduct and Fair Reporting of Clinical Trials." *JAMA,* 1999, 282:1766–68.

45. Bodenheimer, T. "Uneasy Alliance—Clinical Investigators and the Pharmaceutical Industry." *The New England Journal of Medicine,* 2000, 342:1539–44.

46. Huston, P. "Redundancy, Disaggregation, and the Integrity of Medical Research." *Lancet,* April 13, 1996, 347(9007):1024–26.

47. Bodenheimer, op. cit.

48. Hotz, R.L. "Secrecy is often the price of medical research funding." *Los Angeles Times,* May 18, 1999, A-2, 21.

49. Angell, M. "Is Academic Medicine for Sale?" *The New England Journal of Medicine,* May 18, 2000, 342:1516–18.

50. Ibid.

51. Sussman, op. cit.

52. Wazana, A. "Physicians and the pharmaceutical industry: is a gift ever just a gift?" *JAMA,* 2000, 283(3):373–80.

53. *Physicians' Desk Reference,* 54th Edition, Montvale, N.J.: Medical Economics Company, 2000.

54. Cohen and Insel, "The Physicians' Desk Reference. Problems and possible improvements," op. cit.

55. Cohen, "Adverse drug effects, compliance, and the initial doses . . . ," op. cit.

56. Cohen, "Dose discrepancies between the Physicians' Desk Reference . . . ," op. cit.

57. Cohen, "Ways To Minimize Adverse Drug Reactions . . . ," op. cit.

58. Cohen, "Adverse Drug Reactions: Effective Low-Dose Therapies for Older Patients," op. cit.

59. Mullen, W.H., Anderson, I.B., Kim, S.Y., Blanc, P.D., and Olson, K.R. "Incorrect overdose management advice in the Physicians' Desk Reference." *Annals of Emergency Medicine,* 1997, 29(2): 255–61.

60. Gebhart, F. "Is Standard Dosing to Blame for Adverse Drug Reactions?" *Drug Therapy,* Jan. 17, 2000, 34.

61. Food and Drug Administration. Postmarketing Safety of Sildenafil Citrate (Viagra). Summary of Reports of Death in Viagra Users Received from Marketing (Late March) through Mid-November 1998. FDA Web site: http://www.fda.gov/cder/consumerinfo/viagra/safety3.htm

62. Cauchon, D. "FDA Advisors Tied to Industry: Approval Process Riddled with Conflicts of Interest." *USA Today,* Sept. 25, 2000.

63. Moore et al., op. cit.

260

64. *Dickinson's FDA Review,* Sept. 2000, 7:11. Reductions compared times between 1994–95 and 1998–99.

65. Wolfe, S. "FDA medical officers report lower standards permit dangerous drug approvals." *Worst Pills, Best Pills News,* Jan. 1999;5:7–8.

66. Wood A.J. "The safety of new medicines: the importance of asking the right questions." Editorial in *JAMA,* May 12, 1999, 281(18):1753–4.

67. Ibid.

68. Woosley, R.L., Chen, Y., Freiman, J.P., and Gillis, R.A. "Mechanism of the Cardiotoxic Actions of Terfenadine." *JAMA,* 1993, 269(12):1532–6.

69. Moore, T.J. "The FDA in Crisis." *Boston Globe,* Sun., April 2, 2000.

70. Moore, T.J., Psaty, B.M., Furberg, C.D., op. cit.

71. Riva, C. "Consequences of Medical Err—16,000 Swiss Sick from Medicine—Who Is at Fault? The Pharmaceutical Industry or the One Who Writes the Prescription? A New Law Will Oblige Doctors Mention the Side Effects of Medicine." *Dimanche,* April 2, 2000.

72. Angell, "Is Academic Medicine for Sale?" op. cit.

73. Weiss, R. "Correctly Prescribed Drugs Take Heavy Toll." *Washington Post,* Wed., April 15, 1998, A–1, 8.

74. Willman, D. "3 Lawmakers Question FDA on Diabetes Pill Approval: Letter by House Democrats Asks Why Rezulin Was Kept on Market Despite Deaths. Issues Go to 'Heart of Public's Confidence.'" *Los Angeles Times,* Wed., Dec. 23, 1998:A-22.

75. Sulkowski, M.S., Thomas, D.L., Chaisson, R.E., and Moore, R.D. "Hepatotoxicity associated with antiretroviral therapy in adults infected with human immunodeficiency virus and the role of hepatitis C or B virus infection." *JAMA,* Jan. 5, 2000, 283(1):74–80.

76. Neergaard, L. (Associated Press). "Some AIDS Patients Are Hit by Disfiguring Fat Deposits: FDA Says Protease Inhibitor Drugs Are Suspected As a Cause. High Levels of Cholesterol Are Also Reported." *Philadelphia Inquirer,* Mon., June 15, 1998, A-2.

77. Wolfe, S.M., editor. "Sudden Deaths Reported with Pimozide (Orap)." *Worst Pills, Best Pills News,* Public Citizen Health Research Group, Nov., 1999, 5:87.

78. Draganov, P., Durrence, H., Cox, C., and Reuben, A. "Alcohol-Acetaminophen Syndrome: Even Moderate Social Drinkers Are at Risk." *Postgraduate Medicine,* 2000, 107:189–195.

79. "Psychosis due to abrupt discontinuation of an oral contraceptive." *Primary Psychiatry,* Nov. 1999, 6:20.

80. Bynum, R. (Associated Press). "Antibiotic Linked to Stomach Disorder in Infants." *San Diego Union-Tribune,* Fri., Dec. 17, 1999, A-21.

81. Roan, S. "Study Links Breast Cancer, Hormone Use." *Los Angeles Times,* Wed., Jan. 26, 2000, A-1, 15.

82. Associated Press. "Maker of Fen-Phen Paid for Articles: Lawsuit Says Wyeth Hid Dangers Linked to Weight-Loss Drug." *San Diego Union-Tribune,* May 25, 1999.

83. Wolfe, S.M., editor. "New Adverse Reaction Warning: Liver Toxicity with Prostate Cancer Drug Flutamide (Eulexin)." *Worst Pills, Best Pills News,* Public Citizen Health Research Group, Nov. 1999, 5:88.

84. Food and Drug Administration. "Trovan Associated with Liver Injury and Death." Revised Labeling Confirmation to Pfizer, Inc., May 17, 2000, FDA Web site.

85. Page, J., and Henry, D. "Consumption of NSAIDs and the Development of Congestive Heart Failure in Elderly Patients—an Unrecognized Public Health Problem." *Archives of Internal Medicine,* 2000, 160:777–84.

86. de Abajo, F.J., Rodriguez, L.A., and Montero, D. "Association between selective serotonin reuptake inhibitors and upper gastrointestinal bleeding: population based case-control study." *BMJ,* Oct. 23, 1999, 319(7217):1106–9.

87. Maugh, T.H. "Beta-Blockers Linked to Diabetes in Study." *Los Angeles Times,* Mon., April 3, 2000, S3.

88. Lagergren, J., Bergstrom, R., Adami, H.O., Nyren, O. "Association between medications that relax the lower esophageal

sphincter and risk for esophageal adenocarcinoma." *Annals of Internal Medicine,* Aug 1, 2000, 133(3):165–75.

89. Moore et al., "Time to act on drug safety," op. cit.

90. Modell, J.G., Katholi, C.R., Modell, J.D., and DePalma, R.L. "Comparative sexual side effects of bupropion, fluoxetine, paroxetine, and sertraline." *Clinical Pharmacology and Therapeutics,* April 1997, 61(4):476–87.

91. Montejo-Gonzalez, A.L., Llorca, G., Izquierdo, J.A., Ledesma, A., Bousono, M., Calcedo, A., et al. "SSRI-induced sexual dysfunction: fluoxetine, paroxetine, sertraline, and fluvoxamine in a prospective, multicenter, and descriptive clinical study of 344 patients." *Journal of Sex and Marital Therapy,* Fall 1997, 23(3): 176–94.

92. Hirschfeld, R.M. "Management of sexual side effects of antidepressant therapy." *Journal of Clinical Psychiatry.* 1999, 60 Suppl 14:27–30; discussion 31–5.

93. Willman, D. "FDA's expedited drug approvals cost lives." *Los Angeles Times,* Fri., Dec. 29, 2000.

94. Angell, op. cit.

95. Ibid.

96. Sanson-Fisher, R.W., Clover, K. "Compliance in the treatment of hypertension. A need for action." *American Journal of Hypertension,* 1995, 8(10 Pt 2):82S–88S.

97. Feldman, R., Bacher, M., Campbell, N., et al. "Adherence to pharmacologic management of hypertension." *Canadian Journal of Public Health,* 1998, 89(5):I16–8.

98. Roberts, W.C. "The underused miracle drugs: the statin drugs are to atherosclerosis what penicillin was to infectious disease." *American Journal of Cardiology,* 1996, 78:377–8.

99. Avorn, J., Monette, J., Lacour, A., Bohn, R.L., Monane, M., Mogun, H., et al. "Persistence of use of lipid-lowering medications: a cross-national study." *JAMA,* 1998, 279(18):1458–62.

100. Brett, K.M., Madans, J.H. "Use of postmenopausal hormone replacement therapy: estimates from a nationally representative cohort study." *American Journal of Epidemiology,* March 15, 1997, 145(6):536–45.

101. Saver, B.G., Taylor, T.R., Woods, N.F. "Use of hormone replacement therapy in Washington State: is prevention being put into practice?" *Journal of Family Practice,* May 1999, 48(5):364–71.

102 Wood, op. cit.

103. Willman, D. "The Rise and Fall of the Killer Drug Rezulin: People were dying as specialists waged war against their FDA superiors. Patient safety was at stake in the scramble to keep a 'fast-track' pill on the U.S. market." *Los Angeles Times,* Sun., June 4, 2000, A-1, 16–18.

104. William, D. "FDA Minimized Issue of Lotronex's Safety: Times Study Finds Officials Sided with Drug Maker on Regulatory Concerns; Agency Reevaluation Underway." *Los Angeles Times,* Thurs., Nov. 2, 2000:A–1,15.

105. Willman, D. "Blood Pressure Pill OKed Before Study Ended." *Los Angeles Times,* Wed., Jan. 10, 2001.

Chapter 2

1. American Medical Association. *AMA Drug Evaluations, Annual 1993.* Chicago: American Medical Association, 1993.

2. Clark, W.G., Brater, D.C., and Johnson, A.R. *Goth's Medical Pharmacology,* 13th Edition. St. Louis: The C.V. Mosby Company, 1992.

3. Gilman, A.G., Rall, T.W., Nies, A.S., and Taylor, P. *Goodman and Gilman's The Pharmacological Basis of Therapeutics.* New York: Pergamon Press, 1990 and 1996.

4. Martin, E.W. *Hazards of Medication: A Manual on Drug Interactions, Contraindications, and Adverse Reactions with Other Prescribing and Drug Information,* 2nd edition. Philadelphia: J.B. Lippincott Company, 1978.

5. Cohen, J.S. "Dose Discrepancies between the Physicians' Desk Reference and the Medical Literature, and Their Possible Role in the High Incidence of Dose-Related Adverse Drug Events." *Archives of Internal Medicine,* April 9, 2001:161:957–64.

6. Cohen, J.S. Adverse drug effects, compliance, and the initial doses of antihypertensive drugs recommended by the Joint National Committee vs. the Physicians' Desk Reference. *Archives of Internal Medicine,* March 26, 2001;161:880–85.

7. Cohen, J.S. Adverse Drug Reactions: Effective Low-Dose Therapies for Older Patients. *Geriatrics,* Feb. 2000; 55 (2):54–64.

8. Cohen, J.S. Ways to Minimize Adverse Drug Reactions: Individualized Doses and Common Sense Are Key. *Postgraduate Medicine,* Sept. 1999; 106: 163–72.

9–12. Same articles as cited in notes 5–8.

13. Kantor, T.G. "Use of diclofenac in analgesia." *American Journal of Medicine,* 1986, suppl 4B:64–69.

14. Ingemanson, C.A., Carrington, B., Sikstrom, B., and Bjorkman, R. "Diclofenac in the treatment of primary dysmenorrhoea." *Current Therapeutic Research,* 1981, 30(5):632–639.

15. Ciccolunghi, S.N., Chaudri, H.A., and Schubiger, B.I. "The value and results of long-term studies with diclofenac sodium (Voltarol)." *Rheumatology and Rehabilitation,* 1979, suppl 2:100–115.

16. Machtey, I. "Diclofenac in the treatment of painful joints and traumatic tendinitis (including strains and sprains): a brief review." *Seminars in Arthritis and Rheumatism,* 1985, 15(2 Suppl 1):87–92.

17. Duerrigl, T., Vitaus, M., Pucar, I., and Miko, M. "Diclofenac sodium (Voltaren): results of a multi-centre comparative trial in adult-onset rheumatoid arthritis." *Journal of International Medical Research,* 1975, 3:139–144.

18. Mutru, O., Penttila, M., Pesonen, J., Salmela, P., Suhonen, O., and Sonck, T. "Diclofenac sodium (Voltaren) and indomethacin in the ambulatory treatment of rheumatoid arthritis: a double-blind multicentre study." *Scandinavian Journal of Rheumatology,* 1978, (suppl)22:51–56.

19. Ciccolunghi, S.N., Chaudri, H.A., Schubiger, B.I., and Reddrop, R. "Report on a long-term tolerability study of up to two years with diclofenac sodium (Voltaren)." *Scandinavian Journal of Rheumatology,* 1978, (suppl)22:86–96.

20. Ciccolunghi, et al., op. cit.

21. Schneider, L.S. "How Do Physicians Translate Research into Practice?" *Primary Psychiatry,* Aug. 2000, 7: 60–62.

22. Cohen, J.S. "Appropriate Initial Statin Doses for Primary Prevention Patients with Mild-to-Moderate Hypercholesterolemia." Submitted for publication, Feb. 2001.

23. Gebhart, F. "Is Standard Dosing to Blame for Adverse Drug Reactions?" *Drug Therapy*, Jan. 17, 2000, 34.

24. Grady, D. "Too Much of a Good Thing? Doctor Challenges Drug Manual." *New York Times*, Oct. 12, 1999, D1–2.

25. Kessler, D.A., Rose, J.L., Temple, R.J., Schapiro, R., and Griffin, J.P. "Therapeutic-class wars—drug promotion in a competitive marketplace." *The New England Journal of Medicine*, Nov. 17, 1994, 331(20):1350–3.

26. Gebhart, op. cit.

27. Cooper, S.A. "Five Studies on Ibuprofen for Postsurgical Dental Pain." *American Journal of Medicine*, 1984, (7):70–77.

28. Shapiro, S.S. and Diem, K. "The effects of ibuprofen in the treatment of dysmenorrhea." *Current Therapeutic Research*, 1981, 30(3):327–334.

29. Chalmers, T.M. "Clinical experience with ibuprofen in the treatment of rheumatoid arthritis." *Annals of the Rheumatic Diseases*, 1969, 28:513–517.

30. Bloomfield, S.S., Mitchell, J., Bichlmeir, G., and Barden, T.P. "Low dose ibuprofen and aspirin analgesia for postpartum uterine cramps." *Clinical Pharmacology and Therapeutics*, 1983, 33(2):194.

31. Helzner, E.C., Fricke, J., and Cunningham, B.G. "An evaluation of ibuprofen 200mg, ibuprofen 400mg and naproxen 200mg and 400mg in postoperative oral surgery pain." *Clinical Pharmacology and Therapeutics*, 1992, 51(2):122.

32. Brooks, C.D., Schmid, F.R., Biundo, J., Blau, S., Gonzalez-Alcover, R., et al. "Ibuprofen and aspirin in the treatment of rheumatoid arthritis; a cooperative double-blind trial." *Rheumatology and Physical Medicine*, 1970, 10(suppl):48–63.

33. Thompson, M., Bell, D. "Further experience with ibuprofen in the treatment of arthritis." *Rheumatology and Physical Medicine*, 1970, 10(suppl):100–103.

34. Cooper, S.A. "The Relative Efficacy of Ibuprofen in Dental Pain." *Compendium of Continuing Education in Dentistry*, 1987, 8(8):578–597.

35. Singh, G., Ramey, D.R., Morfeld, D., Shi, H., Hatoum, H.T., and Fries, J.F. "Gastrointestinal tract complications of nonsteroidal

anti-inflammatory drug treatment in rheumatoid arthritis. A prospective observational cohort study." *Archives of Internal Medicine,* 1996, 156(14):1530–6.

36. American Medical Association. *AMA Drug Evaluations, Annual 1994.* Chicago: American Medical Association, 1994.

37. Ibid.

38. Wolfe, M.M., Lichtenstein, D.R., Singh, G. "Gastrointestinal toxicity of nonsteroidal anti-inflammatory drugs." *The New England Journal of Medicine,* 1999, 340(24):1888–99.

39. Associated Press, *San Diego Union-Tribune,* December 2, 1998, A-7.

40. Wolfe, S.M. "Update on the Nonsteroidal Anti-inflammatory Drug Celecoxib (Celebrex)." *Worst Pills, Best Pills News,* Public Citizen Health Research Group, Nov. 1999, 5(11):43, 48.

41. Celebrex Package Insert. Searle & Co., 1999.

42. Ibid.

43. Bensen, W.G., Fiechtner, J.J., McMillen, J.I., Zhao, W.W., Yu, S.S., Woods, E.M., et al. "Treatment of osteoarthritis with celecoxib, a cyclooxygenase-2 inhibitor: a randomized controlled trial." *Mayo Clinic Proceedings,* Nov. 1999, 74(11):1095–1105.

44. Ibid.

45. Gale, K. "Drug Doses Frequently Change after Approval." Reuters Health, Mar. 9, 2001: www.reutershealth.com.

Chapter 3

1. Wernicke, J.F., Dunlop, S.R., Dornseif, B.E., Bosomworth, J.C., and Humbert, M. "Low-dose fluoxetine therapy for depression." *Psychopharmacology Bulletin,* 1988, 24(1):183–188.

2. Martin, E.W. *Hazards of Medication: A Manual on Drug Interactions, Contraindications, and Adverse Reactions with Other Prescribing and Drug Information,* 2nd edition. Philadelphia: J.B. Lippincott Company, 1978.

3. Lazarou, J., Pomeranz, B.H., and Corey, P.N. "Incidence of adverse drug reactions in hospitalized patients: a meta-analysis of prospective studies." *JAMA,* April 15, 1998, 279(15):1200–5.

4. Faich, G.A. "Adverse-drug-reaction reporting." *The New England Journal of Medicine,* 1986, 14:1589.

5. Schatzberg, A.F. "Dosing strategies for antidepressant agents." *Journal of Clinical Psychiatry,* 1991:52(5, suppl):14–20.

6. Gram, L.F. "Fluoxetine—review article." *The New England Journal of Medicine,* 1994, 331(20):1354–61.

7. Schatzberg, A.F., Dessain, E., O'Neil, P., Katz, D.L., and Cole, J.O. "Recent studies on selective serotonergic antidepressants: trazodone, fluoxetine, and fluvoxamine." *Journal of Clinical Psychopharmacology,* 1987, 7(6):44S–49S.

8. Rakel, R.E. *Conn's Current Therapy.* Philadelphia: W.B. Saunders Company, 1993.

9. Stewart J.W., Quitkin F.M., and Klein D.F. "The pharmacotherapy of minor depression." *American Journal of Psychotherapy,* 1992, 46(1):23–36.

10. Schatzberg, "Dosing strategies for antidepressant agents," op. cit.

11. Louie, A.K., Lewis, T.B., and Lannon, M.D. "Use of low-dose fluoxetine in major depression and panic disorder." *Journal of Clinical Psychiatry,* 1993, 54(1):435–438.

12. Salzman, C. "Practical considerations in the pharmacologic treatment of depression and anxiety in the elderly." *Journal of Clinical Psychiatry,* 1990, 51:1 (Suppl), 40–43.

13. Cain, J.W. "Poor response to fluoxetine: underlying depression, serotonergic overstimulation, or a 'therapeutic window'?" *Journal of Clinical Psychiatry,* 1992, 53(8):272–277.

14. *Physicians' Desk Reference,* 54th Edition. Montvale, N.J.: Medical Economics Company, 2000.

15. der Kolk, B., Dreyfuss, D., Michaels, M., et al. "Fluoxetine in post-traumatic stress disorder." *Journal of Clinical Psychiatry,* 1994, 55:517–22.

16. Sherman, C. "Long-term side effects surface with SSRIs: insomnia, weight gain, sexual dysfunction emerge as problems affecting compliance." *Clinical Psychiatry News,* 1998, 26(5):1, 8.

17. Pray, D.R., editor. "Pharmacologic Management of Depression: Length of Treatment, Treatment of the Elderly, and Selective

268

Serotonin Reuptake Inhibitors." *Psychiatric Times,* Special Report, August 1993, 1–4.

18. Sherman, op. cit.

19. Fava, M. "Weight gain during short- and long-term treatment with antidepressants." *Primary Psychiatry,* May 2000, 7:28–32. In one study, 25.5 percent of subjects experience weight gains of 7 percent or more.

20. Sherman, op. cit.

21. Modell, J.G., Katholi, C.R., Modell, J.D., and DePalma, R.L. "Comparative sexual side effects of bupropion, fluoxetine, paroxetine, and sertraline." *Clinical Pharmacology and Therapeutics,* April 1997, 61(4):476–87.

22. Waldinger, M.D., Hengeveld, M.W., Zwinderman, A.H., and Olivier, B. "Effect of SSRI antidepressants on ejaculation: a double-blind, randomized, placebo-controlled study with fluoxetine, fluvoxamine, paroxetine, and sertraline." *Journal of Clinical Psychopharmacology,* Aug. 1998, 18(4):274–81.

23. Montejo-Gonzalez, A.L., Llorca, G., Izquierdo, J.A., Ledesma, A., Bousono, M., Calcedo, A., Carrasco, J.L., Ciudad, J., Daniel, E., De la Gandara, J., et al. "SSRI-induced sexual dysfunction: fluoxetine, paroxetine, sertraline, and fluvoxamine in a prospective, multicenter, and descriptive clinical study of 344 patients." *Journal of Sex and Marital Therapy,* Fall 1997, 23(3):176–94.

24. Gitlin, M.J. "Psychotropic medications and their effects on sexual function: diagnosis, biology, and treatment approaches. *Journal of Clinical Psychiatry,* Sept. 1994, 55(9):406–13.

25. "Dutch study attempts to qualify sexual dysfunction profiles among SSRIs." *Primary Psychiatry,* 1997, 4(7):22–3.

26. Pollack, M.H., Reiter, S., and Hammerness, P. "Genitourinary and sexual adverse effects of psychotropic medication." *International Journal of Psychiatry in Medicine,* 1992, 22(4):305 27.

27. Bender, K.J. "New antidepressants: a practical update." *Psychiatric Times,* Feb. 1995, 12(1):2.

28. Hirschfeld, R.M. "Management of sexual side effects of antidepressant therapy." *Journal of Clinical Psychiatry,* 1999, 60 Suppl 14:27–30, discussion 31–5.

29. Ashton, A.K., Rosen, R.C. "Accommodation to serotonin reuptake inhibitor-induced sexual dysfunction." *Journal of Sex and Marital Therapy*, July–Sept. 1998, 24(3):191–2.

30. de Abajo, F.J., Rodriguez, L.A., and Montero, D. "Association between selective serotonin reuptake inhibitors and upper gastrointestinal bleeding: population based case-control study." *BMJ*, Oct. 23, 1999, 319(7217):1106–9.

31. Ginsburg, D.L. "Selective serotonin reuptake inhibitors increase risk of gastrointestinal bleeding." *Primary Psychiatry*, Dec. 1999, 6:15–22.

32. Thapa, P.B., Gideon, P., Cost, T.W., Milam, A.B., and Ray, W.A. "Antidepressants and the risk of falls among nursing home residents." *The New England Journal of Medicine*, Sept. 24, 1998, 339(13):875–82.

33. Sherman, op. cit.

34. "Special Considerations in Switching Antidepressants." *Journal of Clinical Psychiatry—Intercom, the Experts Converse*, Oct. 1995, 1–12.

35. Cohen, J.S. "Dose Discrepancies between the Physicians' Desk Reference and the Medical Literature, and Their Possible Role in the High Incidence of Dose-Related Adverse Drug Events." *Archives of Internal Medicine*, April 9, 2001. Scheduled for publication.

36. Cohen, J.S. and Insel, P.A. "The Physicians' Desk Reference. Problems and possible improvements." *Archives of Internal Medicine*, 1996, 156(13):1375–80.

37. Glenmullen, J. *Prozac Backlash: Overcoming the Dangers of Prozac, Zoloft, Paxil, and Other Antidepressants with Safe, Effective Alternatives*. New York: Simon and Schuster, March 2000.

38. Healy, D. *The Antidepressant Era*. Cambridge, MA: Harvard University Press, Sept. 1997.

39. Hickling, L. Questions Persist concerning Prozac's Role in Suicide Risk. www.drkoop.com Health News, May 11, 2000: www.drkoop.com/dyncon/article.asp?at=N&id=11009.

40. Teicher MH, Glod C, Cole JO. Emergence of intense suicidal preoccupation during fluoxetine treatment. *American Journal of Psychiatry*, 1990;147(2):207.

41. Fitcher, C.G., Jobe, T.H., Braun, B.G. "Does fluoxetine have a therapeutic window?" *Lancet*, 1991; 338.

42. Anderson, G.M., Segman, R.H., King, R.A. "Serotonin and suicidality: the impact of fluoxetine administration. II: Acute neurobiological effects." *Israel Journal of Psychiatry and Related Sciences*, 1995, 32(1):44–50.

43. Lancon C; Bernard D; Bougerol T. [Fluoxetine, akathisia and suicide]. *Encephale*, 1997 May–Jun, 23(3):218–23. Abstract.

44. Liu, C.Y., Yang, Y.Y., Wang, S.J., Fuh, J.L., Liu, H.C. "Fluoxetine-related suicidality and muscle aches in a patient with poststroke depression [letter]." *Journal of Clinical Psychopharmacology*, 1996 Dec. 16(6):466–7.

45. Hickling, op. cit.

46. Jackson, A. "Drug Turned Loving Man into a Killer, Says Judge." *Sydney Morning Herald*, Fri., May 25, 2001.

47. Donovan, S., Clayton, A., Beeharry, M., Jones, S., Kirk, C., Waters, K., et al. "Deliberate self-harm and antidepressant drugs. Investigation of a possible link." *British Journal of Psychiatry*, 2000 Dec. 177:551–6.

48. Gram, op. cit.

49. Louie et al., op. cit.

50. Rakel, op. cit.

51. Cain, op. cit.

52. Schatzberg, "Dosing strategies for antidepressant agents," op. cit.

53. Ibid.

54. Schatzberg et al., "Recent studies on selective serotonergic antidepressants . . . ," op. cit.

Chapter 4

1. McGinn, D. "Viagra's hothouse." *Newsweek*, Dec. 21, 1998, 44–46.

2. Fenichel, R.R. Open letter to David Willman, LA Times reporter, posted Dec. 29, 2000, www.fenichel.net/la_times.htm.

3. Gunter, B. "Viagra Deaths Scrutinized." *Public Citizen*, Nov.–Dec. 1998, 18(6):1, 7.

4. Leland, J. "Not quite Viagra nation." *Newsweek,* Oct. 26, 1998, 68.

5. Food and Drug Administration. Postmarketing Safety of Silde-nafil Citrate (Viagra). Summary of Reports of Death in Viagra Users Received from Marketing (Late March) through Mid-November 1998. FDA Web site: http://www.fda.gov/cder/consumerinfo/viagra/safety3.htm

6. Leland, op. cit.

7. Azarbal, B., Mirocha, J., Shah, P.K., Cercek, B., and Kaul, S. "Adverse Cardiovascular Events Associated with the Use of Viagra." *Journal of the American College of Cardiology,* 2000, 35 (Suppl A): 553A–554A.

8. Moore, T.J., Psaty, B.M., and Furberg, C.D. "Time to act on drug safety." *JAMA,* May 20, 1998, 279(19):1571–3.

9. Dickinson, J.G. *Dickinson's FDA Review,* March 2000, 7(3):13–14.

10. Melmon, K.L., Morrelli, H.F., Hoffman, B.B., and Nierenberg, D.W. *Melmon and Morrelli's Clinical Pharmacology: Basic Principles in Therapeutics,* 3rd edition. New York: McGraw-Hill, Inc., 1993.

11. Schneider, L.S. "How Do Physicians Translate Research into Practice?" *Primary Psychiatry,* Aug. 2000, 7:60–62.

12. Neergaard, L. (Associated Press). "Doctors ordered: Read the drug label. FDA chief says warnings ignored." *San Diego Union-Tribune,* Tues., Dec. 12, 2000, A-5.

13. Willman, D., Anderson, N. "Rezulin's Swift Approval, Slow Removal Raises Issues." *Los Angeles Times,* Mar. 23, 2000: A–1, A–16.

14. Cohen, J.S. "Should Patients Be Given a Low Test Dose of Viagra Initially?" *Drug Safety,* July 2000, 23:1–10.

15. Malozowski, S., and Sahlroot, J.T. "Hemodynamic effects of sildenafil." *The New England Journal of Medicine,* 2000:343.

16. Viagra package insert. Pfizer Labs, a division of Pfizer Inc. New York: May 1998, Nov. 1998, June 1999, Sept. 1999, and Jan. 2000.

17. Goldstein I., Lue, T.F., Padma-Nathan, H., Rosen, R.C., Steers, W.D., and Wicker, P.A. "Oral sildenafil in the treatment of erectile dysfunction. Sildenafil Study Group." *The New England Journal of Medicine,* 1998, 338(20):1397–404.

18. Morales, A., Gingell, C., Collins, M., Wicker, P.A., and Osterloh,

I.H. "Clinical safety of oral sildenafil (Viagra) in the treatment of erectile dysfunction." *International Journal of Impotence Research,* 1998, 10:69–74.

19. Cohen, J.S. "Is the Product Information on Sildenafil (Viagra) Adequate to Facilitate Optimal Therapeutics and to Minimize Adverse Events?" *Annals of Pharmacotherapy,* March 2001: Scheduled for publication.

20. Food and Drug Administration, op. cit.

21. Azarbal et al., op. cit.

22. Rosenblatt, R.A. "FDA Issues New Warnings on Hazards of Viagra Use." *Los Angeles Times,* Nov. 25, 1998, A-1, 14.

23. Wolfe, S.M., Sasich, L., and Barbehenn, E. "Safety of sildenafil citrate." Letter in *Lancet,* 1998, 352(9137):1393.

24. Azarbal et al., op. cit.

25. Feenstra, J., van Drie-Pierik, R.J., Lacle, C.F., and Stricker, B.H. "Acute myocardial infarction associated with sildenafil." *Lancet,* Sept. 19, 1998, 352(9132):957–8.

26. Azarbal et al., op. cit.

27. Cohen, J.S. "Comparison of FDA Reports of Patient Deaths Associated with Sildenafil (Viagra) and with Injectable Alprostadil." *Annals of Pharmacotherapy,* March 2001: Scheduled for publication.

28. Lazarou, J., Pomeranz, B.H., Corey, P.N. "Incidence of adverse drug reactions in hospitalized patients: a meta-analysis of prospective studies." *JAMA,* April 15, 1998, 279(15):1200–5.

29. Leland, op. cit.

30. Arora, R.R., Timoney, M., and Melilli, L. "Acute myocardial infarction after the use of sildenafil." *The New England Journal of Medicine,* 1999, 341(9):700.

Chapter 5

1. Cimons, M. "Scientists Study Gender Gap in Drug Responses." *Los Angeles Times,* Sunday, June 6, 1999, A-1, 8–9.

2. Brandon, M.L., and Weiner, M. "Clinical Investigation of Terfenadine, a Non-Sedating Antihistamine." *Annals of Allergy,* 1980, 44:71–75.

3. Woosley, R.L., Chen, Y., Freiman, J.P., and Gillis, R.A. "Mechanism of the Cardiotoxic Actions of Terfenadine." *JAMA*, 1993, 269(12), 1532–6.

4. Cimons, op. cit.

5. United States General Accounting Office. "Drug Safety: Most Drugs Withdrawn in Recent Years Had Greater Health Risks for Women." GAO-01-286R Drugs Withdrawn from Market, Jan. 19, 2001.

6. Kritz, F.L. "Mars and Venus and Drugs: Sex Differences Create Extra Risks for Women." *Washington Post*, Tues., Feb. 20, 2001, 77.

7. Thurmann, P.A. and Hompesch, B.C. "Influence of gender on the pharmacokinetics and pharmacodynamics of drugs." *International Journal of Clinical Pharmacology and Therapeutics*, Nov. 1998, 36(11):586–90.

8. Kritz, op. cit.

9. Bowman, L. "51% Of U.S. Adults Take 2 Pills or More a Day, Survey Reports." (Scripps Howard News Service) *San Diego Union-Tribune*, Wed., Jan. 17, 2001, A8.

10. Snider, S. "The Pill: 30 Years of Safety Concerns." *U.S. Food and Drug Administration Consumer Magazine*, Dec. 1990.

11. Bottiger, L.E., Boman, G., Eklund, G., and Westerholm, B. "Oral contraceptives and thromboembolic disease: effects of lowering oestrogen content." *Lancet*, May 24, 1980, 1(8178):1097–101.

12. Gillum, L.A., Mamidipudi, S.K., and Johnston, S.C. "Ischemic Stroke Risk with Oral Contraceptives." *JAMA*, 2000; 284:72–70.

13. Bagshaw, S. "The Combined Oral Contraceptive." *Drug Safety*, 1995, 12:91–96.

14. Van Hoften, C., Burger, H., Peeters, P.H., Grobbee, D.E., Van Noord, P.A., and Leufkens, H.G. "Long-term oral contraceptive use increases breast cancer risk in women over 55 years of age: the DOM cohort." *International Journal of Cancer*, Aug. 15, 2000, 87(4):591–4.

15. Beral V. "Mortality among oral-contraceptive users. Royal College of General Practitioners' Oral Contraception Study." *Lancet*, Oct. 8, 1977, 2(8041):727–31.

16. Marks, L. "'Not just a statistic': the history of USA and UK policy over thrombotic disease and the oral contraceptive pill, 1960s-1970s." Social and Science Medicine, 1999, 49 (9):1139–55.

17. Ibid.

18. Ibid.

19. Snider, op. cit.

20. Ibid.

21. Van Hoften et al., op. cit.

22. Burke, W. "Oral Contraceptives and Breast Cancer." *JAMA,* Oct. 11, 2000, 284:1837–38.

23. Shapiro, S.S. and Diem, K. "The effects of ibuprofen in the treatment of dysmenorrhea." *Current Therapeutic Research,* 1981, 30(3): 327–334.

24. American Medical Association. *AMA Drug Evaluations, Annual 1994.* Chicago: American Medical Association, 1994.

25. *Physicians' Desk Reference,* 54th Edition. Montvale, N.J.: Medical Economics Company, 2000.

26. Bensen, W.G., Fiechtner, J.J., McMillen, J.I., Zhao, W.W., et al. "Treatment of osteoarthritis with celecoxib, a cyclooxygenase-2 inhibitor: a randomized controlled trial." *Mayo Clinic Proceedings,* Nov. 1999, 74(11):1095–105.

27. Samsioe G. "The menopause revisited." *International Journal of Gynaecology and Obstetrics,* Oct, 1995, 51(1):1–13.

28. Corson, S.L. "A practical guide to prescribing estrogen replacement therapy." *International Journal of Fertility and Menopausal Studies,* Sept.–Oct. 1995, 40(5):229–47.

29. Samsioe, op. cit.

30. Latner, A.W. "34th Annual Top 200 Drugs." *Pharmacy Times,* 2000, 66(4):16–32.

31. *Physicians' Desk Reference,* op. cit.

32. Dickinson, J.G. "Given estrogenic alternatives, 1 Premarin may be 1 too many." *Dickinson's FDA Review,* Aug. 1997, 4(8):11–12.

33. Brett, K.M., and Madans, J.H. "Use of postmenopausal hormone replacement therapy: estimates from a nationally representative cohort study." *American Journal of Epidemiology,* March 15, 1997, 145(6):536–45.26.

34. McAuliffe, K. "For Hormone Replacement Therapy, One High-Dose Size May Not Fit All." *New York Times*, Sun., June 25, 2000.

35. Ettinger, B. "Personal perspective on low-dosage estrogen therapy for postmenopausal women." *Menopause*, 1999, 6(3):273–6.

36. Ibid.

37. Weinstein, L. "Efficacy of a continuous estrogen-progestin regimen in the menopausal patient." *Obstetrics and Gynecology*, 1987, 69(6):929–32.

38. Greendale, G.A., Reboussin, B.A., Hogan, P., Barnabei, V.M., Shumaker, S., Johnson, S., et al. "Symptom relief and side effects of postmenopausal hormones: results from the Postmenopausal Estrogen/Progestin Interventions Trial." *Obstetrics and Gynecology*, 1998, 92(6):982–8.

39. Ettinger, op. cit.

40. McNagny, S.E. "Prescribing Hormone Replacement Therapy for Menopausal Symptoms." *Annals of Internal Medicine*, 1999, 131: 605–16.

41. American Medical Association. *AMA Drug Evaluations, Annual 1993.* Chicago: American Medical Association, 1993.

42. American Society of Hospital Pharmacists. *American Hospital Formulary Service*, Drug Information 1999. Gerald K. McEvoy, Editor. Bethesda: 1999.

43. Meema, S., Bunker, M.L., and Meema, H.E. "Preventive effect of estrogen on postmenopausal bone loss." *Archives of Internal Medicine*, 1975, 135(11):1436–40.

44. Lindsay, R., Hart, D.M., and Clark, D.M. "The minimum effective dose of estrogen for prevention of postmenopausal bone loss." *Obstetrics and Gynecology*, 1984, 63(6):759–63.

45. Geola, F.L., Frumar, A.M., Tataryn, I.V., Lu, K.H., Hershman, J.M., Eggena, P., Sambhi, M.P., et al. "Biological effects of various doses of conjugated equine estrogens in postmenopausal women." *Journal of Clinical Endocrinology and Metabolism*, 1980, 51(3):620–5.

46. Ettinger, B. "A practical guide to preventing osteoporosis." *Western Journal of Medicine*, 1988, 149(6):691–5.

47. Ettinger, B., Genant, H.K., and Cann, C.E. "Postmenopausal

276

bone loss is prevented by treatment with low-dosage estrogen with calcium." *Annals of Internal Medicine*, Jan. 1987, 106(1): 40–5.

48. Gallagher, J.C., Kable, W.T., and Goldgar, D. "Effect of progestin therapy on cortical and trabecular bone: comparison with estrogen." *American Journal of Medicine*, Feb. 1991, 90(2):171–8.

49. Recker, R.R., Davies, K.M., Dowd, R.M., and Heaney, R.P. "The effect of low-dose continuous estrogen and progesterone therapy with calcium and vitamin D on bone in elderly women. A randomized, controlled trial." *Annals of Internal Medicine*, June 1, 1999, 130(11):897–904.

50. Rochon, P.A., and Gurwitz, J.H. "Prescribing for seniors: Neither Too Much Nor Too Little." *JAMA*, 1999, 282:113–5.

51. Mizunuma, H., Okano, H., Soda, M., Kagami, I., Miyamoto, S., Tokizawa, T., et al. "Prevention of postmenopausal bone loss with minimal uterine bleeding using low dose continuous estrogen/progestin therapy: a 2-year prospective study." *Maturitas*, May 1997, 27(1):69–76.

52. Ettinger, "Personal perspective on low-dosage estrogen . . . ," op. cit.

53. Ibid.

54. Schairer, C., Lubin, J., Troisi, R., Sturgeon, S., Brinton, L., Hoover, R. "Menopausal estrogen and estrogen-progestin replacement therapy and breast cancer risk." *JAMA*, 2000 Jan 26, 283(4):485–91.

55. Breast cancer and hormone replacement therapy: collaborative reanalysis of data from 51 epidemiological studies of 52,705 women with breast cancer and 108,411 women without breast cancer. Collaborative Group on Hormonal Factors in Breast Cancer. *Lancet*, 1997, 350(9084):1047–59.

56. Gapstur, S.M., Morrow, M., Sellers, T.A. "Hormone replacement therapy and risk of breast cancer with a favorable histology: results of the Iowa Women's Health Study." *JAMA*, 1999 Jun 9, 281(22):2091–7.

57. Persson, I., Weiderpass, E., Bergkvist, L., Bergstrom, R., Schairer,

C. "Risks of breast and endometrial cancer after estrogen and estrogen-progestin replacement." *Cancer Causes and Control,* 1999 Aug, 10(4):253–60.

58. Persson, I. "Estrogens in the causation of breast, endometrial and ovarian cancers—evidence and hypotheses from epidemiological findings." *Journal of Steroid Biochemistry and Molecular Biology,* 2000 Nov 30, 74(5):357–64.

59. Rodriguez, C., Patel, A.V., Calle, E.E., Jacob, E.J., Thun, M.J. "Estrogen replacement therapy and ovarian cancer mortality in a large prospective study of U.S. women." *JAMA,* Mar. 21, 2001, 285:1460–65.

60. Genant, H.K., Lucas, J., Weiss, S., Akin, M., Emkey, R., McNaney-Flint, H., Downs, R., Mortola, J., Watts, N., Yang, H.M., et al. "Low-dose esterified estrogen therapy: effects on bone, plasma estradiol concentrations, endometrium, and lipid levels. Estratab/Osteoporosis Study Group." *Archives of Internal Medicine,* Dec. 8–22, 1997, 157(22):2609–15.

61. Prestwood, K.M., Thompson, D.L., Kenny, A.M., Seibel, M.J., Pilbeam, C.C., and Raisz, L.G. "Low dose estrogen and calcium have an additive effect on bone resorption in older women." *Journal of Clinical Endocrinology and Metabolism,* Jan. 1999, 84(1):179–83.

62. Ettinger, B. "Use of low-dosage 17 beta-estradiol for the prevention of osteoporosis." *Clinical Therapeutics,* 1993, 15(6):950–62.

63. Mortola, J., Watts, N., Yang, H.M., et al. "Low-dose esterified estrogen therapy: effects on bone, plasma estradiol concentrations, endometrium, and lipid levels. Estratab/Osteoporosis Study Group." Comments in *Archives of Internal Medicine,* Dec. 8–22, 1997, 157(22):2609–15.

64. Sharp, C.A., Evans, S.F., Risteli, L., Risteli, J., Worsfold, M., and Davie, M.W. "Effects of low- and conventional-dose transcutaneous HRT over 2 years on bone metabolism in younger and older postmenopausal women." *European Journal of Clinical Investigation,* Sept. 1996, 26(9):763–71.

65. Ettinger, B., Genant, H.K., Steiger, P., and Madvig, P. "Low-

278

dosage micronized 17 beta-estradiol prevents bone loss in post-menopausal women." *American Journal of Obstetrics and Gynecology,* Feb. 1992, 166(2):479–88.

66. Schneider, H.P. and Gallagher, J.C. "Moderation of the daily dose of HRT: benefits for patients." *Maturitas,* 1999, 33(Suppl 1):S25–9.

67. Utian, W.H., Burry, K.A., Archer, D.F., Gallagher, J.C., Boyett, R.L., et al. "Efficacy and safety of low, standard, and high dosages of an estradiol transdermal system (Esclim) compared with placebo on vasomotor symptoms in highly symptomatic menopausal patients." *American Journal of Obstetrics and Gynecology,* 1999, 181(1):71–9.

68. Notelovitz, M., Lenihan, J.P., McDermott, M., Kerber, I.J., Nanavati, N., and Arce, J. "Initial 17 beta-estradiol dose for treating vasomotor symptoms." *Obstetrics and Gynecology,* 2000, 95(5): 726–31.

69. De Aloysio, D., Rovati, L.C., Giacovelli, G., Setnikar, I., and Bottiglioni, F. "Efficacy on climacteric symptoms and safety of low dose estradiol transdermal matrix patches. A randomized, double-blind placebo-controlled study." *Arzneimittel-Forschung,* 2000, 50(3):293–300.

70. Speroff, L., Whitcomb, R.W., Kempfert, N.J., Boyd, R.A., Paulissen, J.B., and Rowan, J.P. "Efficacy and local tolerance of a low-dose, 7-day matrix estradiol transdermal system in the treatment of menopausal vasomotor symptoms." *Obstetrics and Gynecology,* 1996, 88(4 Pt 1):587–92.

71. Brett, K.M. and Madans, J.H. "Use of postmenopausal replacement therapy: estimates from a nationally representative cohort study. *American Journal of Epidemiology,* 1977, 145 (6): 536–45.

72. Udoff, L., Langenberg, P., and Adashi, E.Y. "Combined continuous hormone replacement therapy: a critical review." *Obstetrics and Gynecology,* Aug. 1995, 86(2):306–16.

73. Ettinger, B., "Use of low-dosage 17 beta-estradiol . . . ," op. cit.

74. Ettinger, B., "Personal perspective on low-dosage estrogen . . . ," op.cit.

75. Fox, M. (Reuters). "Osteoporosis Drug Cuts Risk of Breast Can-

cer: Incidence Reduced 72%, Study Reports." *San Diego Union-Tribune,* Tues., Feb. 13, 2001, A7.

76. Graham, D.H. and Malaty, H.M. "Alendronate and naproxen are synergistic for development of gastric ulcers." *Archives of Internal Medicine,* Jan. 8, 2001, 161(1):107–10.

77. Hargrove, J. and Osteen, K. "An alternative method of hormone replacement therapy using the natural sex steroids." *Infertility and Reproductive Medicine Clinics of North America,* 1995, 4:653–74.

78. Calhoun, D.A. and Oparil, S. "High blood pressure in women." *International Journal of Fertility and Women's Medicine,* May–June 1997, 42(3):198–205.

79. Hargrove, J., Maxson, W., Wentz, A., and Burnett, L. "Menopausal hormone replacement therapy with continuous daily oral micronized estradiol and progesterone." *Obstetrics and Gynecology,* 1989, 73:606–612.

80. Fitzpatrick, L.A., Good, A. "Micronized progesterone: clinical indications and comparison with current treatments." *Fertility and Sterility,* Sept. 1999, 72(3):389–97.

81. Hargrove et al., "An alternative method of hormone replacement therapy . . . ," op. cit.

82. Cohen, J.S. "Adverse drug effects, compliance, and the initial doses of antihypertensive drugs recommended by the Joint National Committee vs. the Physicians' Desk Reference." *Archives of Internal Medicine,* 2001, 161:880–85.

83. Lewis, C.E. "Characteristics and treatment of hypertension in women: a review of the literature." *American Journal of the Medical Sciences,* April 1996, 311(4):193–9.

84. Israili, Z.H., and Hall, W.D. "Cough and angioneurotic edema associated with angiotensin-converting enzyme inhibitor therapy. A review of the literature and pathophysiology." *Annals of Internal Medicine,* Aug. 1, 1992, 117(3):234–42.

85. Lewis, op. cit.

86. Stolberg, S.G. "FDA Ban Sought on Chemical Used for Cold Remedies." *New York Times,* Oct. 20, 2000.

87. Ose, L., Luurila, O., Eriksson, J., Olsson, A., Lithell, H., and Wid-gren, B. "Efficacy and safety of cerivastatin, 0.2 mg and 0.4 mg, in patients with primary hypercholesterolaemia: a multinational, randomised, double-blind study. Cerivastatin Study Group." *Current Medical Research and Opinion,* 1999, 15(3):228–40.

88. Peters, T.K., Muratti, E.N., and Mehra, M. "Efficacy and safety of fluvastatin in women with primary hypercholesterolaemia." *Drugs,* 1994, 47(Suppl 2):64–72.

89. Leitersdorf, E. "Gender-related response to fluvastatin in pa-tients with heterozygous familial hypercholesterolaemia." *Drugs,* 1994, 47 (Suppl 2):54–8.

90. Inoue, Y., Kaku, K., Okubo, M., Hatao, K., Hatao, M., Kaneko, T., et al. "A multi-centre study of the efficacy and safety of prava-statin in hypercholesterolaemic patients with non-insulin-dependent diabetes mellitus." *Current Medical Research and Opinion,* 1994, 13(4):187–94.

91. Ose et al., op. cit.

92. Welty, F.K. "Cardiovascular Disease and Dyslipidemia in Women." *Archives of Internal Medicine,* Feb. 26, 2001, 161:514–22.

93. Pear, R. [*New York Times* News Service]. "Sex Bias Found in Medical Research." *San Diego Union-Tribune,* Sun., April 30, 2000: A–1, 14.

94. Pear, R. "Sex Differences Called Key in Medical Studies." *The New York Times,* Wed., Apr. 25, 2001: www.nytimes.com.

95. Exploring the Biological Contributions to Human Health: Does Sex Matter? Wizemann, T.M., Pardu, M.L., Editors, Committee on Understanding the Biology of Sex and Gender Differences, Board on Health Sciences Policy, Institute of Medicine, National Academy of Sciences, National Academy Press, 2001.

96. Ettinger, "Personal perspective on low-dosage estrogen . . . ," op. cit.

97. Weinstein, op. cit.

98. Greendale et al., op. cit.

99. Ettinger, "Personal perspective on low-dosage estrogen . . . ," op. cit.

100. McNagny, op. cit.

101. American Medical Association, op. cit.

102. American Society of Hospital Pharmacists, op. cit.

103. American Medical Association, op. cit.

104. American Society of Hospital Pharmacists, op. cit.

105. Ettinger, "Personal perspective on low-dosage estrogen . . . ," op. cit.

106. Ettinger, "A practical guide to preventing osteoporosis," op. cit.

107. Notelovitz et al., op. cit.

108. Schneider and Gallagher, op. cit.

109. De Aloysio et al., op. cit.

110. Speroff et al., op. cit.

Chapter 6

1. "Summary of the Second Report of the National Cholesterol Education Program (NCEP) Expert Panel on Detection, Evaluation, and Treatment of High Blood Cholesterol in Adults." *JAMA*, 1993, 269:3015–23.

2. Roberts, W.C. "The underused miracle drugs: the statin drugs are to atherosclerosis what penicillin was to infectious disease." *American Journal of Cardiology*, 1996, 78:377–8.

3. Latner, A.W. "34th Annual Top 200 Drugs." *Pharmacy Times*, 2000, 66(4):16–32.

4. Wolffenbuttel, B.H., Mahla, G., Muller, D., Pentrup, A., Black, D.M. "Efficacy and safety of a new cholesterol synthesis inhibitor, atorvastatin, in comparison with simvastatin and pravastatin, in subjects with hypercholesterolemia." *Netherlands Journal of Medicine*, April 1998, 52(4):131–7.

5. Nowrocki, J., Weiss, S., et al. "Reduction in LDL Cholesterol by 25% to 60% in Patients with Primary Hypercholesterolemia by Atorvastatin, a New HMG-Co-A Reductase Inhibitor." *Arteriosclerosis, Thrombosis, and Vascular Biology*, 1995, 15:678–682.

6. *Physicians' Desk Reference*, 54th Edition. Montvale, N.J.: Medical Economics Company, 2000.

7. Stolberg, S.G., and Gerth, J. "How research benefits marketing." *New York Times*, Dec. 23, 2000: www.nytimes.com.

282

8. Pfizer Inc. Lipitor Advertisement. *Postgraduate Medicine,* Dec. 2000, 7:47. "72% of patients reached their NCEP LDL-C goal at 10 mg."

9. Wierzbicki, A.S., Lumb, P.J., Semra, Y., Chik, G., Christ, E.R., and Crook, M.A. "Atorvastatin compared with simvastatin-based therapies in the management of severe familial hyperlipi-daemias." *QJM,* July 1999, 92(7):387–94.

10. Bradford, R.H., Shear, C.L., Chremos, A.N., Dujovne, C., Down-ton, M., Franklin, F.A., et al. "Expanded Clinical Evaluation of Lovastatin (EXCEL) study results. I. Efficacy in modifying plasma lipoproteins and adverse event profile in 8245 patients with moderate hypercholesterolemia." *Archives of Internal Medicine,* Jan. 1991, 151(1):43–9.

11. Roberts, op. cit.

12. Avorn, J., Monette, J., Lacour, A., Bohn, R.L., Monane, M., Mogun, H., and LeLorier, J. "Persistence of use of lipid-lowering medications: a cross-national study." *JAMA,* 1998, 279(18):1458–62.

13. Insull W. "The problem of compliance to cholesterol altering therapy." *Journal of Internal Medicine,* April 1997, 241(4):317–25.

14. Simons, L.A., Levis, G., and Simons, J. "Apparent discontinuation rates in patients prescribed lipid-lowering drugs." *Medical Journal of Australia,* 1996, 164(4):208–11.

15. Duerksen, S. "2 San Diego Scientists Raise Questions about Cholesterol-Cutting Drugs." *San Diego Union-Tribune,* Mon., May 28, 2001:A1, 18.

16. Ibid.

17. Ibid.

18. Wolfe, S.M. "FDA safety office recommends warning about liver failure with cholesterol lowering statin drugs." *Worst Pills, Best Pills News,* Public Citizen Research Group, Jan. 2001, 7(1):8.

19. Chang, J, Green, L. Food and Drug Administration Memorandum. United States Department of Health and Human Services, May 1, 2000: www.fda.gov/ohrms/pocket/ac/00/backgrd/3622b1b_pm_safety_review.pdf.

20. Roberts, W.C. "The rule of 5 and the rule of 7 in lipid-lowering by statin drugs." *American Journal of Cardiology,* 1997, 80: 106–7.

21. Barnett, B.P. Department of Health and Human Services, Food

and Drug Administration, Public Hearing on FDA Regulation of Over-the-Counter Products, June 29, 2000, page 151: www.fda. gov/ohrms/dockets/dockets/00n1256/tr0002a_0012.pdf.

22. Summary of the Second Report of the National Cholesterol Education Program (NCEP) Expert Panel on Detection, Evaluation, and Treatment of High Blood Cholesterol in Adults. *JAMA*, 1993;269:3015–23.

23. Hulley, S.B., Grady, D., Browner, W.S. "Statins: Underused by Those Who Would Benefit—but Caution Is Needed for Young People at Low Risk of Cardiovascular Disease." *British Medical Journal*, 2000, 321:971–72.

24. Jauhar, S. "Weighing Benefits and Risks of Statins." *New York Times*, Sept. 5, 2000.

25. Summary of the Second Report of the National Cholesterol Education Program (NCEP) Expert Panel, op. cit.

26. Wierzbicki, A.S., Lumb, P.J., Chik, G., and Crook, M.A. "High-density lipoprotein cholesterol and triglyceride response with simvastatin versus atorvastatin in familial hypercholesterolemia." *American Journal of Cardiology*, 2000, 86(5):547–9.

27. Roberts, op. cit.

28. Fager, G., Wiklund, O. "Cholesterol reduction and clinical benefit. Are there limits to our expectations?" *Arteriosclerosis, Thrombosis, and Vascular Biology*, 1997, 17(12):3527–33.

29. Lewis, S.J., Moye, L.A., Sacks, F.M., Johnstone, D.E., Timmis, G., Mitchell, J., et al. "Effect of pravastatin on cardiovascular events in older patients with myocardial infarction and cholesterol levels in the average range. Results of the Cholesterol and Recurrent Events (CARE) trial." *Annals of Internal Medicine*, 1998, 129(9):681–9.

30. "West of Scotland Coronary Prevention Study: identification of high-risk groups and comparison with other cardiovascular intervention trials." *Lancet*, Nov. 16, 1996, 348(9038):1339–42.

31. Bristol-Myers Squibb. Advisory Committee Meeting Briefing Book for the Rx to OTC Switch of Pravachol (Pravastatin Sodium). Joint Meeting of Nonprescription Drugs Advisory Committee and Endocrinologic and Metabolic Drugs Advisory Committee,

FDA Web site, 2000: www.fda.gov/ohrms/dockets/ac/00/backgrd/3622b2a_part1.pdf.

32. Nonprescription Mevacor, FDA Advisory Committee Background Information, FDA Web site, June 2000: www.fda.gov/ohrms/dockets/ac/00/backgrd/3622b1b.pdf.

33. Aoki, N. "Drug Makers' Influence Pondered." *The Boston Globe,* May 31, 2001: www.boston.com/globe/

34. *Physicians' Desk Reference,* 54th Edition. Montvale, N.J.: Medical Economics Company, 2000.

35. Steinhagen-Thiessen, E. "Comparative efficacy and tolerability of 5 and 10 mg simvastatin and 10 mg pravastatin in moderate primary hypercholesterolemia." Simvastatin Pravastatin European Study Group. *Cardiology,* 1994, 85(3–4):244–54.

36. Itoh, T., Matsumoto, M., Hougaku, H., Handa, N., Tsubakihara, Y., Yamada, Y., et al. "Effects of low-dose simvastatin therapy on serum lipid levels in patients with moderate hypercholesterolemia: a 12-month study." The Simvastatin Study Group. *Clinical Therapeutics,* 1997; 19(3):487–97.

37. Antonicelli, R., Onorato, G., Pagelli, P., Pierazzoli, L., and Paciaroni, E. "Simvastatin in the treatment of hypercholesterolemia in elderly patients." *Clinical Therapeutics,* 1990, 12(2):165–71.

38. Steinhagen-Thiessen, op. cit.

39. *Physicians' Desk Reference,* op. cit.

40. Graedon, J., and Graedon, T. "The People's Pharmacy" column. *Los Angeles Times,* March 6, 2000.

41. Graedon, J., and Graedon, T. "The People's Pharmacy" column. *Los Angeles Times,* Mon., May 21, 2000, S-2,6.

42. Graedon, J., and Graedon, T. "The People's Pharmacy" column. *Los Angeles Times,* Mon., Jan. 15, 2001, S2.

43. Davignon, J., Hanefeld, M., Nakaya, N., Hunninghake, D.B., Insull, W., Jr., and Ose, L. "Clinical efficacy and safety of cerivastatin: summary of pivotal phase IIb/III studies." *American Journal of Cardiology,* 1998; 82(4B):32J–39J.

44. Betteridge, D.J. "International multicentre comparison of cerivastatin with placebo and simvastatin for the treatment of patients with primary hypercholesterolaemia." International

Cerivastatin Study Group. *International Journal of Clinical Practice,* 1999, 53(4):243–50.

45. Arca, M., Vega, G.L., and Grundy, S.M. "Hypercholesterolemia in postmenopausal women: metabolic defects and response to low-dose lovastatin." *JAMA,* 1994, 271(6):453–9.

46. Rubinstein, A., Lurie, Y., Groskop, I., Weintrob, M. "Cholesterol-lowering effects of a 10 mg daily dose of lovastatin in patients with initial total cholesterol levels 200 to 240 mg/dl (5.18 to 6.21 mmol/liter)." *American Journal of Cardiology,* Nov. 1, 1991, 68(11):1123–6.

47. Ibid.

48. Duerksen, S., op. cit.

49. Gotto, A.M. "Coronary heart disease in the United States: the scope of the problem." *Lipid management in clinical practice: report from the National Lipid Education Council,* 1996, 1(2):4.

Chapter 7

1. Feldman, R., Bacher, M., Campbell, N., et al. "Adherence to pharmacologic management of hypertension." *Canadian Journal of Public Health,* 1998, 89(5):I16–8.

2. Alderman, M.H., Madhavan, S., and Cohen, H. "Antihypertensive Drug Therapy. The effect of JNC criteria on prescribing patterns and patient status through the first year." *American Journal of Hypertension,* 1996, 9(5):413–8.

3. Tomlinson, B. "Optimal dosage of ACE inhibitors in older patients." *Drugs and Aging,* 1996, 9(4):262–73.

4. Flack, J.M., Novikov, S.V., and Ferrario, C.M. "Benefits of adherence to anti-hypertensive drug therapy." *European Heart Journal,* 1996, 17 (Suppl A): 16–28.

5. "Hypertension Management Today," Albert Einstein College Of Medicine, Office Of Continuing Medication, June 1996, 1(1), 1–14.

6. Rakel, R.E. *Conn's Current Therapy 1995.* Philadelphia: W.B. Saunders Company, 1995.

7. Elliott, W.J., Maddy, R., Toto, R., and Bakris, G. "Hypertension in Patients with Diabetes." *Postgraduate Medicine,* 2000, 107:29–38.

8. Sorrentino, M.J. "Turning up the heat on hypertension. It's time to be more aggressive in finding and treating this silent killer." *Postgraduate Medicine,* May 1, 1999, 105(5):82–4, 89–93.

9. Curzen, N., Purcell, H. "Matching the treatment to the patient in hypertension." *Practitioner,* 1997, 241(1572):152–6.

10. Cohen, J.S. "Adverse drug effects, compliance, and the initial doses of antihypertensive drugs recommended by the Joint National Committee vs. the Physicians' Desk Reference." *Archives of Internal Medicine,* 2001, 161:880–85.

11. "The Sixth Report of the Joint National Committee on Prevention, Detection, Evaluation, and Treatment of High Blood Pressure." *Archives of Internal Medicine,* 1997, 157:2413–46.

12. Cohen, J.S. and Insel, P.A. "The *Physicians' Desk Reference,* Problems And Possible Improvements." *Archives of Internal Medicine,* 1996, 156:1375–80.

13. Connelly, D.P., Rich, E.C., Curley, S.P., and Kelly, J.T. "Knowledge resource preferences of family physicians." *Journal of Family Practice,* 1990, 30(3):353–9.

14. Hyman, D.J. and Pavlik, V.N. "Self-Reported Hypertension Treatment Practices Among Primary Care Physicians." *Archives of Internal Medicine,* 2000, 160:2281–86.

15. Gibson, G.R. "Enalapril-induced cough." *Archives of Internal Medicine,* Dec. 1989, 149(12):2701–3.

16. Kubota, K., Kubota, N., Pearce, G.L., and Inman, W.H. "ACE-inhibitor-induced cough, an adverse drug reaction unrecognised for several years: studies in prescription-event monitoring." *European Journal of Clinical Pharmacology,* 1996, 49(6):431–7.

17. Heckbert, S.R., Longstreth, W.T., Jr., Psaty, B.M., Murros, K.E., Smith, N.L., Newman, A.B., et al. "The association of antihypertensive agents with MRI white matter findings and with Modified Mini-Mental State Examination in older adults." *Journal of the American Geriatrics Society,* Dec. 1997, 45(12):1423–33.

18. Havlik, R.J. "Antihypertensive drugs, brain structure, and cognitive function: more research is necessary." *Journal of the American Geriatrics Society,* Dec. 1997, 45(12):1529–31.

19. Pahor, M., Psaty, B.M., Alderman, M.H., Applegate, W.B.,

Williamson, J.D., et. al. "Health outcomes associated with calcium antagonists compared with other first-line antihypertensive therapies: a meta-analysis of randomized controlled trials." *Lancet*, Dec. 9, 2000;356(9246):1949–54.

20. Psaty, B.M., Smith, N.L., Siscovick, D.S., Koepsell, T.D., Weiss, N.S., Heckbert, S.R., et al. "Health outcomes associated with antihypertensive therapies used as first-line agents. A systematic review and meta-analysis." *JAMA*, March 5, 1997, 277(9):739–45.

21. Gurwitz, J.H., Everitt, D.E., Monane, M., Glynn, R.J., Choodnovskiy, I., Beaudet, M.P., and Avorn, J. "The impact of ibuprofen on the efficacy of antihypertensive treatment with hydrochlorothiazide in elderly persons." *Journals of Gerontology*. Series A, Biological Sciences and Medical Sciences, March 1996, 51(2):M74–9.

22. Gurwitz, J.H., Avorn, J., Bohn, R.L., Glynn, R.J., Monane, M., and Mogun, H. "Initiation of antihypertensive treatment during nonsteroidal anti-inflammatory drug therapy." *JAMA*, Sept. 14, 1994, 272(10):781–6.

Chapter 8

1. Smucker, W.D. and Kontak, J.R. "Adverse drug reactions causing hospital admission in an elderly population: experience with a decision algorithm." *Journal of the American Board of Family Practice*, April–June, 1990, 3(2):105–9.

2. Montamat, S.C., Cusack, B.J., and Vestal, R.E. "Management of drug therapy in the elderly." *New England Journal of Medicine*, Aug. 3, 1989, 321(5):303–9.

3. Brawn, L.A. and Castleden, C.M. "Adverse drug reactions. An overview of special considerations in the management of the elderly patient." *Drug Safety*, Nov.–Dec., 1990, 5(6):421–35.

4. Gibian, T. "Rational drug therapy in the elderly or How not to poison your elderly patients." *Australian Family Physician*, Dec. 1992, 21(12):1755–60.

5. Wolfe, S.M. and Hope, R.E. *Worst Pills, Best Pills II: The Older Adult's Guide to Avoiding Drug-Induced Death or Illness*. Washington, D.C.: Public Citizen's Health Research Group, 1993.

6. Rochon, P.A., Anderson, G.M., Tu, J.V., Gurwitz, J.H., Clark, J.P.,

Shear, N.H., and Lau, P. "Age- and gender-related use of low-dose drug therapy: the need to manufacture low-dose therapy and evaluate the minimum effective dose." *Journal of the American Geriatrics Society*, Aug. 1999, 47(8):954–9.

7. Tinkelman, D., Falliers, M., et al. "Efficacy and safety of fexofenadine in fall seasonal allergic rhinitis." *Journal of Allergy and Clinical Immunology*, 1996, 97(1):1009.

8. Brandon, M.L., Weiner, M. "Clinical Studies of Terfenadine [Seldane] in Seasonal Allergic Rhinitis." *Arzneimittel-Forschung/Drug Research*, 1982; 32(11):1204–5.

9. Brandon, M.L., Weiner, M. "Clinical Investigation of Terfenadine, a Non-Sedating Antihistamine." *Annals of Allergy*, 1980; 44:71–75.

10. Lauritsen, K., Andersen, B.N., Laursen, L.S., Hansen, J., Havelund, T., Eriksen, J., et al. "Omeprazole 20 mg three days a week and 10 mg daily in prevention of duodenal ulcer relapse; double-blind comparative trial." *Gastroenterology*, March 1991, 100(3): 663–9.

11. Lauritsen, K., Andersen, B.N., Havelund, T., Laursen, L.S., and Hansen, J. "Effect of 10 mg and 20 mg omeprazole daily on duodenal ulcer: double-blind comparative trial." *Alimentary Pharmacology and Therapeutics*, 1989, 3(1): 59–67.

12. Langman, J.S., Henry, D.A., and Ogilvie, A. "Ranitidine and Cimetidine for Duodenal Ulcer." *Scandinavian Journal of Gastroenterology*, 1981, 69(suppl):115–7.

13. Berstad, A., Kett, K., Aadland, E., Carlsen, E., Frislid, K., et al. "Treatment of Duodenal Ulcer with ranitidine, a New Histamine H2-Receptor Antagonist." *Scandinavian Journal of Gastroenterology*, 1980, 15(5):637–9.

14. Dobrilla, G., Barbara, L., Bianchi-Porro, G., Felder, M., Mazzacca, G., et al. "Placebo Controlled Studies with Ranitidine in Duodenal Ulcer." *Scandinavian Journal of Gastroenterology*, 1981, 69(suppl):101–105.

15. Dobrilla, G., de Pretis, G., Felder, M., and Chilovi, F. "Endoscopic double-blind controlled trial of ranitidine vs placebo in the short-term treatment of duodenal ulcer." *Hepato-Gastroenterology*, 1981, 28(1):49–52.

16. Cloud, M.L., Offen, W.W., Matsumoto, C. "Healing and subsequent recurrence of duodenal ulcer in a clinical trial comparing nizatidine 300-mg and 100-mg evening doses and placebo in the treatment of active duodenal ulcer." *Current Therapeutics and Research, Clinical Experience,* 1989, 45(3):359–367.

17. Dyck, W.P., Cloud, M.L., Offen, W.W., Matsumoto, C., Chernish, S.M. "Treatment of duodenal ulcers in the United States." *Scandinavian Journal of Gastroenterology,* 1987, 22(suppl 136):47–55.

18. Samanta, A., Nahass, D., and Habba, S. "Efficacy of nizatidine: a new H2 receptor antagonist in the treatment of duodenal ulcer; a dose response study." *American Journal of Gastroenterology,* 1986, 81(9):852.

19. Savarino, V., Mela, G.S., Zentilin, P., Bonifacino, G., Moretti, M., Valle, F., and Celle, G. "Low bedtime doses of H2-receptor antagonists for acute treatment of duodenal ulcers." *Digestive Diseases and Sciences,* 1989, 34(7):1043–46.

20. Fiorucci, S., Clausi, G.G., Cascetta, R., Farinelli, M.F., Pelli, M.A., and Morelli, A. "Effects of low and high doses of famotidine and ranitidine on nocturnal gastric pH." *Digestive Diseases and Science,* 1986, 31(Suppl 10):393S.

21. Feldman, R., Bacher, M., Campbell, N., et al. "Adherence to pharmacologic management of hypertension." *Canadian Journal of Public Health,* 1998, 89(5):I16–8.

22. Alderman, M.H., Madhavan, S., and Cohen, H. "Antihypertensive Drug Therapy. The effect of JNC criteria on prescribing patterns and patient status through the first year." *American Journal of Hypertension,* 1996, 9(5):413–8.

23. Tomlinson B. "Optimal dosage of ACE inhibitors in older patients." *Drugs and Aging,* 1996, 9(4):262–73.

24. Flack, J.M., Novikov, S.V., and Ferrario, C.M. "Benefits of adherence to anti-hypertensive drug therapy." *European Heart Journal,* 1996, 17(Suppl A):16–20.

25. "High Blood Pressure Said to Increase Cognitive Decline in the Elderly." *Primary Psychiatry,* 2000, 7:20–22.

26. Wolfe, M.M., Lichtenstein, D.R., and Singh, G. "Gastrointestinal

toxicity of nonsteroidal anti-inflammatory drugs." *New England Journal of Medicine,* 1999, 340(24):1888–99.

27. Wolfe, S.M., op. cit.

28. Bensen, W.G., Fiechtner, J.J., McMillen, J.I., Zhao, W.W., Yu, S.S., Woods, E.M., et al. "Treatment of osteoarthritis with celecoxib, a cyclooxygenase-2 inhibitor: a randomized controlled trial." *Mayo Clinic Proceedings,* Nov. 1999, 74(11):1095–105.

29. Bowman, L. "51% Of U.S. Adults Take 2 Pills or More a Day, Survey Reports" (Scripps Howard News Service). *San Diego Union-Tribune,* Wed., Jan. 17, 2001, A8.

30. Williams, R.D. "Medications and older adults." *FDA Consumer Magazine,* Sept.–Oct. 1997.

31. Ibid.

32. Page, J. and Henry, D. "Consumption of NSAIDs and the Development of Congestive Heart Failure in Elderly Patients—an Unrecognized Public Health Problem." *Archives of Internal Medicine,* 2000, 160:777–84.

33. Ibid.

34. Kolata, Gina. "What ails elderly often prescribed" (New York Times News Service). *San Diego Union-Tribune,* July 27, 1994, A-1, 20.

35. Oh, V.M. "Multiple medication: problems of the elderly patient." *International Dental Journal,* Dec. 1991, 41(6):348–58.

36. Gurwitz, J.H., Field, T.S., Avorn, J., McCormick, D., Jain, S., Eckler, M., et al. "Incidence and preventability of adverse drug events in nursing homes." *American Journal of Medicine,* 2000, 109(2):87–94.

Chapter 9

1. Peck, C., Barr, W., Benet, L., Collins, J., Desjardins, R., Furst, D., et al. "Opportunities for integrating of pharmacokinetics, pharmacodynamics, and toxicokinetics in rational drug development." *Journal of Clinical Pharmacology,* 1994, 34:111–9.

2. Angell, M. "Is Academic Medicine for Sale?" *The New England Journal of Medicine,* May 18, 2000, 342(20):1516–18.

3. Ibid.

4. Ibid.

5. Ibid.

6. Leibowitz, J. "Is Academic Medicine for Sale?" *The New England Journal of Medicine,* Aug. 17, 2000, 343(7):509.

7. Ross, L.F. "Is Academic Medicine for Sale?" *The New England Journal of Medicine,* Aug. 17, 2000, 343:509.

8. Davidson, R.A. "Source of funding and outcome of clinical trials." *Journal of General Internal Medicine,* May–June 1986, 1(3): 155–8.

9. Bero, L.A. and Rennie, D. "Influences on the quality of published drug studies." *International Journal of Technology Assessment in Health Care,* Spring 1996, 12(2):209–37.

10. Stelfox, H.T., Chua, G., O'Rourke, K., and Detsky, A.S. "Conflict of interest in the debate over calcium-channel antagonists." *New England Journal of Medicine,* Jan. 8, 1998, 338(2):101–6.

11. Friedberg, M., Saffran, B., Stinson, T.J., Nelson, W., and Bennett, C.L. Evaluation of conflict of interest in economic analyses of new drugs used in oncology. *JAMA,* Oct. 20, 1999, 282(15):1453–7.

12. Steiner, I. and Wirguin, I. "Multiple sclerosis—in need of a clinical reappraisal." *Medical Hypotheses,* 2000, 54:99–106.

13. (Associated Press). "Teen's death prompts U.S. look at big research deals." *Los Angeles Times,* Wed., Aug. 16, 2000, A-9.

14. Chalmers, I. "Underreporting research is scientific misconduct." *JAMA,* March 9, 1990, 263(10):1405–8.

15. Bodenheimer, T. "Uneasy Alliance—Clinical Investigators and the Pharmaceutical Industry." *The New England Journal of Medicine,* 2000, 342:1539–44.

16. Ibid.

17. Rochon P.A., Gurwitz, J.H., Simms, R.W., Fortin, P.R., Felson, D.T., Minaker, K.L., et al. "A study of manufacturer-supported trials of nonsteroidal anti-inflammatory drugs in the treatment of arthritis." *Archives of Internal Medicine,* Jan. 24, 1994, 154(2): 157–63.

292

18. Bodenheimer, op. cit.

19. Moore, T.J., Psaty, B.M., and Furberg, C.D. "Time to act on drug safety." *JAMA,* May 20, 1998, 279(19):1571–3.

20. Chalmers, op. cit.

21. Bodenheimer, op. cit.

22. Ibid.

23. Hotz, R.L. "Secrecy is often the price of medical research funding." *Los Angeles Times,* May 18, 1999, A-2, 21.

24. Ibid.

25. Bodenheimer, op. cit.

26. Hotz, op. cit.

27. Ibid.

28. Bodenheimer, T. and Collins, R. "The Ethical Dilemmas of Drugs, Money, Medicine." *Seattle Times,* Wed., Mar. 15, 2001: Web site.

29. Bodenheimer, "Uneasy Alliance . . . ," op. cit.

30. Ibid.

31. Bodenheimer et al. "The Ethical Dilemmas . . . ," op. cit.

32. Adams, C. "A Determined Doctor Writes a New Prescription for Drug Research." *The Wall Street Journal,* Dec. 10, 1999, B1, 4.

33. Ray, W.A., Griffin, M.R., and Avorn, J. "Evaluating Drugs after Their Approval for Clinical Use." *The New England Journal of Medicine,* 1993, 329:2029–32.

34. Stolberg, S.G., and Gerth, J. "How research benefits marketing." *New York Times,* Dec. 23, 2000, www.nytimes.com.

35. Garattini, S. and Liberati, A. "The risk of bias from omitted research: evidence must be independently sought and free of economic interests." *British Medical Journal,* 2000, 321:845–6.

36. Adams, op. cit.

37. Ibid.

38. Ibid.

39. Sasich, L.D., Lurie, P., and Wolfe, S.M. "The Drug Industry's Performance in Finishing Post-Marketing Research (Phase 4) Studies: a Public Citizen's Health Research Group Reported." Public Citizen Health Research Group, April 13, 2000, www.citizen.org/hrg/PUBLICATIONS/1520.htm.

40. Wolfe, S.M. "Dangerous Gap in the Drug Safety System: Companies May Be Failing to Keep Their Post-Marketing Research Promises." *Worst Pills, Best Pills News,* June 2000, 6:41–42.

41. Warner, S. "The Politics of Prescription Drugs." *Philadelphia Inquirer,* July 30, 2000, E-1, 3.

42. Gerth, J. and Stolberg, S.G. "Drug Industry Has Ties to Groups with Many Different Voices." *New York Times,* Oct. 5, 2000: www.nytimes.com.

43. Gale, K. "Drug Doses Frequently Change after Approval." Reuters Health, Mar. 9, 2001, www.reutershealth.com.

44. Peck, C.C. "Drug development: improving the process." *Food Drug Law Journal,* 1997, 52:163–7.

45. Rennie, D. "Fair Conduct and Fair Reporting of Clinical Trials." *JAMA,* 1999, 282:1766–68.

46. Huston, P. "Redundancy, Disaggregation, and the Integrity of Medical Research." *Lancet,* April 13, 1996, 347(9007):1024–26.

47. Rennie, op. cit.

48. Bodenheimer, "Uneasy Alliance . . . ," op. cit.

49. Larkin M. "Whose article is it anyway?" *Lancet,* July 10, 1999, 354(9173):136.

50. Ibid.

51. Brennan, T.A. "Buying editorials." *The New England Journal of Medicine,* 1994, 331:673–5.

52. Flanagin, A., Carey, L.A., Fontanarosa, P.B., Phillips, S.G., Pace, B.P., Lundberg, G.D., and Rennie, D. "Prevalence of articles with honorary authors and ghost authors in peer-reviewed medical journals." *JAMA,* July 15, 1998, 280(3):222–4.

53. Stolberg, S.G. "Scientists Often Mum about Ties to Industry." *New York Times,* Wed., Apr. 25, 2001: www.nytimes.com.

54. Brennan, op. cit.

55. Bodenheimer et al. "Ethical Dilemmas . . . ," op. cit.

56. (Associated Press). "Maker of Fen-Phen Paid for Articles: Lawsuit Says Wyeth Hid Dangers Linked to Weight-Loss Drug." *San Diego Union-Tribune,* May 25, 1999.

57. Ibid.

58. Ibid.

294

59. Associated Press. "Diet Drug Firm Accused of Funding Favorable Articles." *Los Angeles Times,* May 24, 1999.

60. McKenzie, J. "A Conflict of Interest? Doctors Walk Fine Line When Taking Gifts from Drug Companies." ABC News, Feb. 17, 2000, www.ABC.com.

61. Ibid.

62. ABC Evening News, May 30, 2000.

63. Wazana, A. "Physicians and the pharmaceutical industry: is a gift ever just a gift?" *JAMA,* 2000, 283(3):373–80.

64. Ibid.

65. Ibid.

66. Wazana, A. "Gifts to physicians from the pharmaceutical industry." *JAMA,* 2000, 283:2656–8.

67. Norton, J.W. "Is Academic Medicine for Sale?" *The New England Journal of Medicine,* Aug. 17, 2000, 343:508.

68. Wazana, A. "Gifts to physicians from the pharmaceutical industry." op. cit.

69. McKenzie, op. cit.

70. Tenery, R. "Gifts to physicians from the pharmaceutical industry." *JAMA,* 2000, 283:2656–8.

71. Cohen, J.S. and Insel, P.A. "The Physicians' Desk Reference. Problems and possible improvements." *Archives of Internal Medicine,* 1996, 156(13):1375–80.

72. Cohen, J.S. "Ways To Minimize Adverse Drug Reactions: Individualized Doses and Common Sense Are Key." *Postgraduate Medicine,* Sept. 1999, 106:163–72.

73. Cohen and Insel, op. cit.

74. Cohen, J.S. "Adverse drug effects, compliance, and the initial doses of antihypertensive drugs recommended by the Joint National Committee vs. the Physicians' Desk Reference." *Archives of Internal Medicine,* 2001, 161:880–85.

75. Cohen, J.S. "Dose Discrepancies between the Physicians' Desk Reference and the Medical Literature, and Their Possible Role in the High Incidence of Dose-Related Adverse Drug Events." *Archives of Internal Medicine,* April 9, 2001: Scheduled for publication.

76. Cohen, "Ways to Minimize Adverse Drug Reactions . . . ," op. cit.

77. Cohen, J.S. "Adverse Drug Reactions: Effective Low-Dose Therapies for Older Patients." *Geriatrics,* Feb. 2000, 55(2):54–64.

78. Mullen, W.H., Anderson, I.B., Kim, S.Y., Blanc, P.D., and Olson, K.R. "Incorrect overdose management advice in the Physicians' Desk Reference." *Annals of Emergency Medicine,* 1997, 29(2): 255–61.

79. Ibid.

80. Cohen and Insel, op. cit.

81. (Associated Press). "Report Rips Nation's Health Care System." *San Diego Union-Tribune,* Fri., March 2, 2001, A18.

82. Monmaney, T. "Medical Journal Urges Curbs on Researcher Ties to Drug Firms." *Los Angeles Times,* Thurs., May 18, 2000, A-31.

83. Ibid.

84. Altman, L.K. "New England Journal of Medicine Names Third Editor in a Year." *New York Times,* May 12, 2000.

85. Ibid.

86. Monmaney, T. "Top Medical Journal Admits 19 Lapses of Ethics Policy." *Los Angeles Times,* Thurs., Feb. 25, 2000, A-1, 22.

87. Ibid.

88. Fontana, R.J., McCashland, T.M., Benner, K.G., Appelman, H.D., Gunartanam, N.T., Wisecarver, J.L., et al. "Acute liver failure associated with prolonged use of bromfenac leading to liver transplantation." The Acute Liver Failure Study Group. *Liver Transplantation and Surgery,* Nov, 1999, 5(6):480–4.

89. Moore, T.J. "The FDA in Crisis." *Boston Globe,* Sun., April 2, 2000.

90. Ibid.

91. Ibid.

92. Wood, A.J. "The safety of new medicines: the importance of asking the right questions." Editorial in *JAMA,* May 12, 1999, 281(18):1753–4.

93. Susman, N. "Benzodiazepines: Do They Still Have a Clinical Role in the Treatment of Panic Disorder?" *Primary Psychiatry,* March 2001;8(3):32–36.

94. *Physicians' Desk Reference,* 54th Edition. Montvale, N.J.: Medical Economics Company, 2000.

95. Ibid.

96. Use of Zyban As an Aid to Relapse Prevention. Letter, Sept. 26, 1998. GlaxoWellcome, Research Triangle Park, North Carolina.

97. Dobson, R. "Antismoking drug comes under scrutiny for deaths." *British Medical Journal,* Feb. 24, 2001;322:452.

98. *Physicians' Desk Reference,* 54th Edition. Montvale, N.J.: Medical Economics Company, 2000.

99. Ibid.

100. Rossner, S., Sjostrom, L., Noack, R., Meinders, A.E., Noseda, G. "Weight loss, weight maintenance, and improved cardiovascular risk factors after 2 years treatment with orlistat for obesity." European Orlistat Obesity Study Group. *Obesity Research,* 2000 Jan, 8(1):49–61.52.

101. Hauptman, J., Lucas, C., Boldrin, M.N., Collins, H., Segal, K.R. "Orlistat in the long-term treatment of obesity in primary care settings." *Archives of Family Medicine,* 2000 Feb, 9(2):160–7.

102. Lucas, K.H., Kaplan-Machlis, B. "Orlistat—a Novel Weight Loss Therapy." *Annals of Pharmacotherapy,* Mar. 2001;35(3):314–28.

103. Judd, J. "Truth in Advertising? FDA Says Many Prescription Drug Ads Are Deceptive." ABC News, Jan. 3, 2001, www.ABCNews.com.

104. Ibid.

105. Ibid.

106. Wolfe, S. "New Research on Direct-to-Consumer Prescription Drug Advertising." *Worst Pills, Best Pills News,* Jan. 2000;6(1):5.

107. Judd, op. cit.

108. Ibid.

109. Neergaard, L. (Associated Press). Aspirin claims cost Bayer $1 million. *San Diego Union-Tribune,* Wed., Jan. 12, 2000:A8.

110. Tramer, M.R. "Aspirin, like all other drugs, is a poison." *British Medical Journal,* 2000, 321:1170–71.

111. Meade, T.W. and Brennan, P.J. "Determination of who may derive most benefit from aspirin in primary prevention: subgroup results from a randomised controlled trial." *British Medical Journal,* July 1, 2000, 321(7252):13–7.

112. Neergaard, op. cit.

113. Dickinson, J,G. "Medical marketers 'laughing at FDA.'" *Dickinson's FDA Review,* July 1999, 6(7):4–7.

114. Ibid.

115. Ibid.

116. Wolfe, op. cit.

117. Dickinson, op. cit.

118. DeAngelis, C.D. "The Plight of Academic Health Centers." *JAMA,* 2000, 283:2438–39.

119. Gerth, Stolberg, op. cit.

120. Kessler, D.A., Rose, J.L., Temple, R.J., Schapiro, R., Griffin, J.P. "Therapeutic-class wars—drug promotion in a competitive marketplace." *The New England Journal of Medicine,* Nov. 17, 1994, 331(20):1350–3.

121. Ibid.

122. Angell, M. "The Pharmaceutical Industry—To Whom Is It Accountable?" *The New England Journal of Medicine,* June 22, 2000, 342(25):1902–04.

123. Ibid.

124. Ibid.

125. Ibid.

Chapter 10

1. Dickinson, J.G. "Medical marketers 'laughing at FDA.'" *Dickinson's FDA Review,* July 1999, 6(7):4–7.

2. Angell, M. "Is Academic Medicine for Sale?" *The New England Journal of Medicine,* Aug. 17, 2000, 343:510.

3. Peck, C., Barr, W., Benet, L., Collins, J., Desjardins, R., Furst, D., et al. "Opportunities for integrating of pharmacokinetics, pharmacodynamics, and toxicokinetics in rational drug development." *Journal of Clinical Pharmacology,* 1994, 34:111–9.

4. Bensen, W.G., Fiechtner, J.J., McMillen, J.I., Zhao, W.W., Yu, S.S., Woods, E.M., et al. "Treatment of osteoarthritis with celecoxib, a cyclooxygenase-2 inhibitor: a randomized controlled trial." *Mayo Clinic Proceedings,* Nov. 1999, 74(11):1095–105.

5. (Associated Press). "Tests urged of pills' role in vehicular fatalities." *San Diego Union-Tribune,* Wed., Jan. 19, 2000, A-6.

6. Weiler, J.M., Bloomfield, J.R., Woodworth, G.G., Grant, A.R., Layton, T.A., Brown, T.L., et al. "Effects of fexofenadine, diphenhydramine, and alcohol on driving performance. A randomized, placebo-controlled trial in the Iowa driving simulator." *Annals of Internal Medicine,* March 7, 2000, 132(5):354–63.

Chapter 11

1. Kaplan, S. "Events shake doctor's faith in drug safety." *Los Angeles Times,* Sun., June 4, 2000, A17.

2. Willman, D. "The Rise and Fall of the Killer Drug Rezulin: People were dying as specialists waged war against their FDA superiors. Patient safety was at stake in the scramble to keep a 'fast-track' pill on the U.S. market." *Los Angeles Times,* Sun., June 4, 2000, A-1,16–18.

3. Ibid.

4. Ibid.

5. Ibid.

6. Ibid.

7. Moore, T.J. "The FDA in Crisis." *Boston Globe,* Sun., April 2, 2000.

8. Kaplan, op. cit.

9. Willman, op. cit.

10. Ibid.

11. Moore, op. cit.

12. Willman, Ibid.

13. Willman, D. "Key FDA Aide In Rezulin Case Resigns." *Los Angeles Times,* Thurs., Oct. 19, 2000, A-8.

14. Willman, "The Rise and Fall of the Killer Drug Rezulin . . . ," op. cit.

15. Woosley, R.L. "Drug Labeling Revisions—Guaranteed to Fail?" *JAMA,* Dec. 20, 2000, 284(23):3047.

16. Moore, op. cit.

17. Willman, "Key FDA Aide In Rezulin Case Resigns," op. cit.

18. Willman, D. "FDA Official Says Lessons Have Been Learned from Rezulin." *Los Angeles Times,* Sun., June 4, 2000, A16.

19. Willman, D. "Fears Grow over Delay in Removing Rezulin: Five

FDA Physicians Say the Lives of Diabetes Patients Are at Stake." *Los Angeles Times,* Fri., Mar. 10, 2000:A1,18,19.

20. Willman, "The Rise and Fall of the Killer Drug Rezulin . . . ," op. cit.

21. Ibid.

22. Ibid.

23. Willman, D., Anderson, N. "Rezulin's Swift Approval, Slow Removal Raises Issues." *Los Angeles Times,* Mar. 23, 2000: A–1, A–16.

24. Kaplan, op. cit.

25. Kaplan, op. cit.

26. Willman, "The Rise and Fall of the Killer Drug Rezulin," op. cit.

27. Ibid.

28. Ibid.

29. Ibid.

30. Moore, op. cit.

31. Kaplan, op. cit.

32. Willman, D. "FDA's expedited drug approvals cost lives." *Los Angeles Times,* Fri., Dec. 29, 2000.

33. Ibid.

34. Grady, D. "After Diabetes Drug, New Questions for the FDA." *New York Times,* March 23, 2000.

35. Ibid.

36. Willman, D. "FDA Panel Not Told of Drug's Ill Effects." *Los Angeles Times,* Fri., Dec. 18, 1998, A12.

37. *Physicians' Desk Reference,* 52nd Edition. Montvale, N.J.: Medical Economics Company, 1998.

38. Willman, "The Rise and Fall of the Killer Drug Rezulin . . . ," op. cit.

39. Lurie, P. and Wolfe, S.M. "FDA Medical Officers Report Lower Standards Permit Dangerous Drug Approvals." *Public Citizen,* Aug. 2000, www.citizen.org.

40. Wolfe, S. "FDA medical officers report lower standards permit dangerous drug approvals." *Worst Pills, Best Pills News,* Jan. 1999, 5:7–8.

41. (Associated Press). "FDA's policy on new drugs is criticized." *San Diego Union-Tribune,* August 26, 1998, A-8.

42. Fenichel, R.R. Letter, Dec. 29, 2000, to David Willman following *Los Angeles Times* article on the FDA: www.fenichel.net/la_times.htm.

43. Lurie and Wolfe, op. cit.

44. Dickinson, J.G. *Dickinson's FDA Review,* Feb. 1999, 6:2.

45. Dickinson, J.G. "More on Lotronex." *Dickinson's FDA Review,* Nov. 2000, 7:4–5.

46. Willman, D. "FDA Minimized Issue of Lotronex's Safety: Times Study Finds Officials Sided with Drug Maker or Regulatory Concerns; Agency Reevaluation Underway." *Los Angeles Times,* Thurs., Nov. 2, 2000, A-1, 15.

47. Ibid.

48. Willman, D. "Blood Pressure Pill OKed Before Study Ended." *Los Angeles Times,* Wed., Jan. 10, 2001.

49. Ibid.

50. Ibid.

51. FDA committee recommends approval for Viagra rival. *British Medical Journal,* April 22, 2000, 320:1094.

52. "Looking Beyond Viagra." *Newsweek,* April 24, 2000, 77–78.

53. Ibid.

54. Lurie and Wolfe, op. cit.

55. "Looking Beyond Viagra," op. cit.

56. Cauchon, D. "FDA Advisors Tied to Industry: Approval Process Riddled with Conflicts of Interest." *USA Today,* Sept. 25, 2000.

57. Ibid.

58. Willman, D. "Scientists who judged pill safety received fees." *Los Angeles Times,* Fri., Oct. 29, 1999, A22.

59. Dickinson, J.G. "Rezulin reviewers see bias in advisory committee." *Dickinson's FDA Review,* Dec, 2000, 7(12):15–16.

60. Gribbin, A. "House investigated panels involved with drug safety." *The Washington Times,* Mon., June 18, 2001: www.washtimes.com.

61. Food and Drug Administration. Herceptin Warning Letter, May 3, 2000:www.fda.gov.

62. "Fifteen Deaths Are Linked to Breast Cancer Drug." *New York Times,* Fri., May 5, 2000.

63. Moore, op. cit.

64. Ibid.

65. Lauritsen, K., Andersen, B.N., Havelund, T., Laursen, L.S., Hansen, J. "Effect of 10 mg and 20 mg omeprazole daily on duodenal ulcer: double-blind comparative trial." *Alimentary Pharmacology and Therapeutics,* 1989, 3(1):59–67.

66. Grady, D. "FDA Pulls a Drug, and Patients Despair." *New York Times,* Jan. 30, 2001, www.nytimes.com.

67. Ibid.

68. Ibid.

69. Ibid.

70. Moore, op. cit.

71. Ibid.

72. Wolfe, S. "Public citizen in the courts: Health Research Group sues the FDA over access to drug information." *Worst Pills, Best Pills News,* March 1999, 4:36.

73. Ibid.

74. Wolfe, "FDA medical officers report lower standards . . . ," op. cit.

75. Willman, "FDA's expedited drug approvals cost lives," op. cit.

76. Ibid.

77. Kolata, G. "Who cares when our drugs fail?" (New York Times News Service). *San Diego Union-Tribune,* Wed., Oct. 15, 1997, E-5.

78. Henney, J. "Better Surveillance Planned." *USA Today,* July 13, 2000.

79. Misbin, R.I. "Rethink Method of Protecting Patients." *USA Today,* Aug. 3, 2000, 18A.

80. Ibid.

81. Honig, P., Phillips, J., and Woodcock, J. Center for Drug Evaluation and Research. U.S. Food and Drug Administration. "How Many Deaths Are Due to Medical Errors?" *JAMA,* 2000, 284: 2187–8.

82. U.S. Government, Department of Health and Human Services, Food and Drug Administration. Requirements on Content and Format of Labeling for Human Prescription Drugs and Biologics: Proposed Rule. Federal Register, Dec. 22, 2000; 65(247): 81081–81124.

Chapter 12

1. Wood, A.J.J., Stein, C.M., and Woosley, R. "Making Medicines Safer: the Need for An Independent Drug Safety Board." *The New England Journal of Medicine,* 1998, 339:1851–54.

2. Moore, T.J., Psaty, B.M., and Furberg, C.D. "Time to act on drug safety." *JAMA,* May 20, 1998, 279(19):1571–3.

3. Wood et al., op. cit.

4. Ibid.

5. Dickinson, J.G. *Dickinson's FDA Review,* March 2000, 7(3):13–14.

6. Bates, D.W. "Drugs and adverse drug reactions: how worried should we be?" *JAMA,* April 15, 1998, 279(15):1216–7.

7. Moore et al., op. cit.

8. Kessler, D.A. "Introducing MedWatch: a New Approach to Reporting Medication and Device Adverse Effects and Product Problems." *JAMA,* 1993, 269:2765–68.

9. Kolata, G. "Who cares when our drugs fail?" (New York Times News Service). *San Diego Union-Tribune,* Wed., Oct. 15, 1997, E-5.

10. Bates, op. cit.

11. Kolate, G., op. cit.

12. Grady, D. "Calculating Safety in Risky World of Drugs." *New York Times,* Wed., March 6, 2001.

13. Ibid.

14. Wood et al., op. cit.

15. Ray, W.A., Griffin, M.R., and Avorn, J. "Evaluating Drugs after Their Approval for Clinical Use." *New England Journal of Medicine,* 1993, 329:2029–32.

16. Neergaard, L. "Doctors ordered: Read the drug label. FDA chief says warnings ignored." (Associated Press). *San Diego Union-Tribune,* Tues., Dec. 12, 2000, A-5.

17. Moore et al., op. cit.

18. Ibid.

19. Ibid.

20. Wolfe, S. "Consumer Alert: False and Misleading Claims for Raloxifene (Evista) by Eli Lilly and Company." *Worst Pills, Best Pills News,* March 1999, 5:18, 23.

21. Avorn, J. "Drug Regulation and Drug Information—Who Should Do What to Whom?" Editorial in *American Journal of Public Health*, 1995, 85:18–19.

22. Hirsh, J. "Is the Dose of Warfarin Prescribed by American Physicians Unnecessarily High?" *Archives of Internal Medicine*, 1987, 47:769–771.

23. Ibid.

24. Hull, R., Hirsh, J., Jay, R., Carter, C., England, C., Gent, M., et al. "Different Intensities of Oral Anticoagulant Therapy in the Long-term Treatment of Proximal Vein Thrombosis." *New England Journal of Medicine*, 1982, 307:1676–1681.

25. Eckman, M.H., Levine, H.J., and Pauker, S.G. "Effect Of Laboratory Variation In The Prothrombin-Time Ratio On The Results Of Oral Anticoagulant Therapy." *The New England Journal of Medicine*, 1993, 329(10):696–70.

26. Ibid.

27. Moore et al., op. cit.

28. Ibid.

29. Wood et al., op. cit.

30. Ibid.

31. Willman, D. 3 Lawmakers Question FDA on Diabetes Pill Approval: Letter by House Democrats Asks Why Rezulin Was Kept on Market Despite Deaths. Issues Go to "Heart of Public's Confidence." *Los Angeles Times*, Wed., Dec. 23, 1998: A-22.

32. Cohen, J.S. "Comparison of FDA Reports of Patient Deaths Associated with Sildenafil (Viagra) and with Injectable Alprostadil." *Annals of Pharmacotherapy*, March 2001;35:285–88.

Chapter 13

1. Avorn J. "The prescription as final common pathway." *International Journal of Technology Assessment in Health Care*, 1995, 11(3):384–90.

2. Somberg, J.C. "The drug development process and clinical practice." Editorial in *Journal of Clinical Pharmacology*, 1990, 30:673.

3. Ross, D. and Bukata, R. "Optimizing prescribing practices, Part 2." *Emergency Medicine & Acute Care Essays,* 1993, 17(1):1–5.

4. Wood, A.J.J., Stein, C.M., and Woosley, R. "Making Medicines Safer: the Need for An Independent Drug Safety Board." *The New England Journal of Medicine,* 1998, 339:1851–54.

5. Woosley, R.L. "Drug Labeling Revisions—Guaranteed to Fail?" *JAMA,* Dec. 20, 2000, 284(23):3047–49.

6. *Physicians' Desk Reference,* 54th Edition. Montvale, N.J.: Medical Economics Company, 2000.

7. Ibid.

8. Hedenmalm, K., Spigset, O. "Peripheral sensory disturbances related to treatment with fluoroquinolones." *Journal of Antimicrobial Chemotherapy,* 1996; 37(4):831–7.

9. Graedon, J. and Graedon, T. "The People's Pharmacy." *Los Angeles Times,* Mon., Dec. 4, 2000, S-2.

10. Cohen, J.S. "The One-Size Dose Does Not Fit All: Look beyond the guidelines of drug manufacturers." *Newsweek,* Dec. 6, 1999, 92.

11. Honein, M.A., Paulozzi, L.J., Himelright, I.M., Lee, B., Cragan, J.D., Patterson, L., et al. "Infantile hypertrophic pyloric stenosis after pertussis prophylaxis with erythromcyin: a case review and cohort study." *Lancet,* Dec. 18–25, 1999, 354(9196):2101–5.

12. de Abajo, F.J., Rodriguez, L.A., and Montero, D. "Association between selective serotonin reuptake inhibitors and upper gastrointestinal bleeding: population based case-control study." *British Medical Journal,* Oct. 23, 1999, 319(7217):1106–9.

13. Cotterchio, M., Kreiger, N., Darlington, G., and Steingart, A. "Antidepressant medication use and breast cancer risk." *American Journal of Epidemiology,* May 15, 2000, 151(10):951–7.

14. Modai, I., Hirschmann, S., Rava, A., Kurs, R., Barak, P., Lichtenberg, P., and Ritsner, M. "Sudden death in patients receiving clozapine treatment: a preliminary investigation." *Journal of Clinical Psychopharmacology,* June 2000, 20(3):325–7.

15. Schneider, L.S. "Mellaril Gets Clocked." *Primary Psychiatry,* 2000, 7:24–25.

16. Moore, T.J., Psaty, B.M., and Furberg, C.D. "Time to act on drug safety." *JAMA,* May 20, 1998, 279(19):1571–3.

17. Wolfe, S.M., and Hope, R.E. *Worst Pills, Best Pills II: The Older Adult's Guide to Avoiding Drug-Induced Death or Illness.* Washington, D.C.: Public Citizen's Health Research Group, 1993.

18. George, C.F. "Adverse drug reactions and secrecy." *British Medical Journal,* 1992, 304(23):1328.

19. Braddock, C.H., Edwards, K.A., Hasenberg, N.M., Laidley, T.L., and Levinson, W. "Informed Decision Making in Outpatient Practice: Time to Get Back to Basics." *JAMA,* 1999, 282:2313–20.

20. Marshall, E. "Financial Conflict: Universities Puncture Modest Regulatory Trial Balloon." *Science Magazine,* March 16, 2001, 2060.

21. "Leading NIH-Funded Medical Schools Agree on Guidelines That Would Strengthen Conflict of Interest Policies of Virtually All Schools, Hospitals, and Research Institutes." Proposal submitted to National Medical College Association. Harvard Medical School Office of Public Affairs. February 8, 2001.

22. Martin, E.W. *Hazards of Medication: A Manual on Drug Interactions, Contraindications, and Adverse Reactions with Other Prescribing and Drug Information,* 2nd edition. Philadelphia: J.B. Lippincott Company, 1978.

23. Dalen, J.E. "Health Care in America: the Good, the Bad, and the Ugly." *Archives of Internal Medicine,* 2000, 160:2573–76.

24. Kolata, G. "Who cares when our drugs fail?" (New York Times News Service). *San Diego Union-Tribune,* Wed., Oct. 15, 1997, E-1, 5.

25. American Medical Association. *AMA Drug Evaluations, Annual 1993.* Chicago: American Medical Association, 1993.

26. Naranjo, C.A., Busto, U., Sellers, E.M., Sandor, P., Ruiz, I., Roberts, E.A., et al. "A method for estimating the probability of adverse drug reactions." *Clinical Pharmacology and Therapeutics,* Aug. 1981, 30(2):239–45.

26. Brodell, R.T. "Do More Than Discuss That Unusual Case." *Postgraduate Medicine,* 2000, 108:19–21.

28. Melmon, K.L., Morrelli, H.F., Hoffman, B.B., and Nierenberg, D.W. *Melmon and Morrelli's Clinical Pharmacology: Basic Principles in Therapeutics,* 3rd edition. New York: McGraw-Hill, Inc., 1993.

29. DeAngelis, C.D. "The Plight of Academic Health Centers." *JAMA,* 2000, 283:2438–39.

Chapter 14

1. Cimons, M. "Scientists Study Gender Gap in Drug Responses." *Los Angeles Times,* Sunday, June 6, 1999, A-1, 8–9.

2. Gilman, A.G., Rall, T.W., Nies, A.S., Taylor, P. *Goodman and Gilman's The Pharmacological Basis of Therapeutics.* New York: Pergamon Press, 1990 and 1996.

3. Gebhart, F. "Is Standard Dosing to Blame for Adverse Drug Reactions?" *Drug Therapy,* Jan. 17, 2000, 34.

4. Cohen, J.S. "Ways To Minimize Adverse Drug Reactions: Individualized Doses and Common Sense Are Key." *Postgraduate Medicine,* Sept. 1999, 106:163–72.

5. Grady, D. "Too Much of a Good Thing? Doctor Challenges Drug Manual." *New York Times,* Oct. 12, 1999, D1–2.

6. "Are You Taking Too Much Medicine: the Standard Recommended Starting Dose May Not Be the Best Choice for You." *Consumer Reports,* March 2000, 62–63.

7. *Physicians' Desk Reference,* 54th edition. Montvale, N.J.: Medical Economics Company, 2000.

8. Ibid.

9. Graedon, J. and Graedon, T. "The People's Pharmacy." *Los Angeles Times,* Mon. Jan. 8, 2001, S2.

10. Sjoqvist, F. and Bertilsson, L. "Clinical pharmacology of antidepressant drugs: Pharmacogenetics." *Advances in Biochemical Psychopharmacology,* 1984, 39:359–372.

11. *United States Pharmacopeia, Drug Information (USP DI): Drug Information for the Health Care Professional.* Taunton, MA: Rand McNally, 1994.

12. Hall, S.S. "Claritin and Schering-Plough: a Prescription for Profit." *New York Times,* March 11, 2001, www.nytimes.com.

13. Metz, D.C., Pisegna, J.R., Fishbeyn, V.A., Benya, R.V., Feigenbaum, K.M., Koviack, P.D., and Jensen, R.T. "Currently used doses of omeprazole in Zollinger-Ellison symdrome are too high." *Gastroenterology,* 1992, 103:1498–1508.

14. Marcuard, S.P., Albernaz, L., Khazanie, P.G. "Omeprazole therapy causes malabsorption of cyanocobalamin (vitamin B_{12}). *Annals of Internal Medicine,* Feb. 1, 1994, 120(3):211–5.

15. Keuthen, N.J., Cyr, P., Ricciardi, J.A., Minichiello, W.E., Buttolph, M.L., Jenike, M.A. "Medication withdrawal symptoms in obsessive-compulsive disorder patients treated with paroxetine [letter]." *Journal of Clinical Psychopharmacology*, Jun. 1994, 14(3):206–7.

16. Pacheco, L., Malo, P., Aragues, E., Etxebeste, M. "More cases of paroxetine withdrawal syndrome [letter]." *British Journal of Psychiatry*, Sep. 1996, 169(3):384.

17. *Physicians' Desk Reference*, 54th Edition. Montvale, N.J.: Medical Economics Company, 2000.

18. *Physicians' Desk Reference*. Ibid.

19. Grady, D. "Calculating Safety in Risky World of Drugs." *New York Times*, Wed., March 6, 2001.

20. Ibid.

21. Wolfe, S. *Worst Pills, Best Pills*, Nov. 2000, 6:87.

22. Pyke, R.E. "Paroxetine withdrawal syndrome." Letter in *American Journal of Psychiatry*, Jan. 1995, 152(1):17.

23. Keuthen, N.J., Cyr, P., Ricciardi, J.A., Minichiello, W.E., Buttolph, M.L., and Jenike, M.A., op. cit.

24. Pacheco, L., Malo, P., Aragues, E., and Etxebeste, M., op. cit.

25. Barr, L.C., Goodman, W.K., and Price, L.H. "Physical symptoms associated with paroxetine discontinuation." Letter in *American Journal of Psychiatry*, Feb. 1994, 151(2):289.

26. "Psychosis due to abrupt discontinuation of an oral contraceptive." *Primary Psychiatry*, Nov. 1999, 6:20.

27. Melmon, K.L., Morrelli, H.F., Hoffman, B.B., and Nierenberg, D.W. *Melmon and Morrelli's Clinical Pharmacology: Basic Principles in Therapeutics*, 3rd edition. New York: McGraw-Hill, Inc., 1993.

28. Graham, D.Y., Malaty, H.M. "Alendronate and Naproxen Are Synergistic for Development of Gastric Ulcers." *Archives of Internal Medicine*, 2001, 161:107–10.

29. American Medical Association Council on Ethical and Judicial Affairs. *Code of Medical Ethics*, 1998–1999 edition. American Medical Association, Chicago, IL.

30. Braddock, C.H., 3rd, Fihn, S.D., Levinson, W., Jonsen, A.R., and Pearlman, R.A. "How doctors and patients discuss routine clini-

cal decisions. Informed decision making in the outpatient setting." *Journal of General Internal Medicine,* June 1997, 12(6): 339–45.

31. Little, P., Everitt, H., Williamson, I., Warner, G., Moore, M., Gould, C., et al. "Preferences of Patients for Patient Centered Approach to Consultation in Primary Care: Observational Study." *British Medical Journal,* Feb. 24, 2001, 322:1–7.

32. American Society of Hospital Pharmacists. *American Hospital Formulary Service, Drug Information 1993, 1994, 1995, and 1996.* Gerald K. McEvoy, editor. Bethesda: 1993–1996.

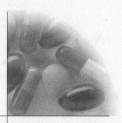

Index

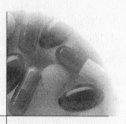

About the Author

JAY S. COHEN, M.D., is an associate professor of family and preventive medicine and of psychiatry, voluntary, at the University of California, San Diego, where he teaches medical students and staff. From 1980 to 1991, he was a member of the Department of Internal Medicine of the Naval Regional Medical Center at Balboa Hospital, San Diego. In 1972–73 he was on staff at UCLA.

Dr. Cohen initially practiced general and community medicine, pain research at UCLA, then psychiatry and psychopharmacology (the expertise of psychiatric drugs). His primary interest has always been pharmacology—the optimal use of medications in order to maximize effectiveness and minimize side effects.

In 1990, after twenty years of clinical experience, Dr. Cohen left private practice due to a disabling medical condition that rendered him housebound and bedridden from 1995 through 1999. During this time, as his condition allowed, he pursued his research in the underlying causes of the high incidence of medication side effects. Without any funding or staff, he has been able to publish many articles in the medical literature and, in 1998, *Make Your Medicine Safe: How to Prevent Side Effects from the Drugs You Take* (Avon Books). Dr. Cohen's work has been highlighted in *The New York Times, Consumer Reports, Woman's Day,* and many other publications.

In 1998, Dr. Cohen realized that one of his medical problems was erythromelalgia, a rare, painful neurovascular disorder affecting blood flow to the limbs. He became a member, and subsequently a board member, of The Erythromelalgia Association (TEA) (www. erythromelalgia.com). Working with other TEA members and communicating with the few experts in the world, Dr. Cohen organized and published a major review article to inform patients and physicians how to diagnose and treat this perplexing disorder. After trying scores of treatments himself, he discovered a new treatment that has markedly improved his health.

Dr. Cohen lives with his wife and son in San Diego.